eat to lose, eat to win

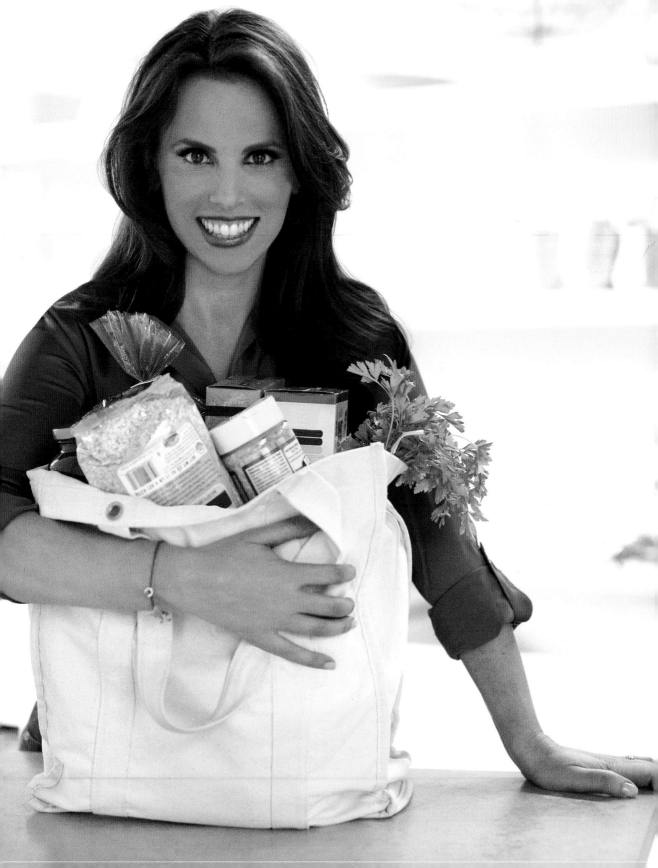

eat to lose, eat to win

your grab-n-go action plan
for a slimmer, healthier you

Rachel Beller, M.S., R.D.

WM

WILLIAM MORROW
An Imprint of HarperCollinsPublishers

This book is written as a source of information only. The information contained in this book should by no means be considered a substitute for the advice of a qualified medical professional, who should always be consulted before beginning any new diet, exercise, or other health program.

All efforts have been made to ensure the accuracy of the information contained in this book as of the date published. The authors and the publisher expressly disclaim responsibility for any adverse effects arising from the use or application of the information contained herein.

The author sometimes receives product samples for consideration and independent analysis but is not paid to represent any of the products featured in this book.

Calorie counts are approximate; they may vary, depending on the brand and variety you buy.

FOOD AUTOPSY is a trademark of Beller Nutritional Institute, LLC.

HarperCollins books may be purchased for educational, business, or sales promotional use. For information please write: Special Markets Department, HarperCollins Publishers, 10 East 53rd Street, New York, NY 10022.

FIRST EDITION

Designed by Kris Tobiassen

Library of Congress Cataloging-in-Publication Data has been applied for.

ISBN 978-0-06-223181-9

13 14 15 16 17 ID/QG 10 9 8 7 6 5 4 3 2 1

To my parents,
the loving forces of my life;

my four kids,
for putting a smile on my face
each and every day;

and my husband,
who is my best friend

contents

PART 3

shop yourself skinny

PART 4

just the facts

foreword
by sheryl crow

Here's why I absolutely love Rachel Beller and why I'm so excited that her book, *Eat to Lose, Eat to Win,* is *finally* out. (It's about time, Rachel!)

This is not just another diet book, and Rachel is not just another dietitian. Rachel is so much more. Her advice isn't just for people trying to lose weight, it's also for people like me who want to eat "defensively." It's life-changing advice—literally. And she actually makes it fun.

My story certainly didn't begin in a fun way. Far from it. I can still hear the three words from my oncologist that completely altered my life: "You have cancer."

When I heard that, I sat in disbelief. "But I'm super-fit. I'm only forty-two. I'm a good person." At that moment I knew I'd never look at life the same way again.

That was February 2006. I had gone in for a routine mammogram, which showed some suspect calcifications. Those aren't unusual for someone my age, so I was told to come back in six months. But my obstetrician urged me to have a needle biopsy right away, just to make sure the calcifications weren't anything to worry about. The odds of it being cancer were only 5 percent, but the look on the face of my surgical oncologist, Dr. Kristi Funk, told me that my cancer was invasive.

The early days of my diagnosis are a strange kind of wash in my mind. I did what I always do when facing a challenge: I got down to fixing it. I met a recommended oncologist, Philomena McAndrew, and began schooling myself on cancer, as if it were a course I could master. I surrounded myself with friends and family, creating a fortress in which I could feel scared and sad and confused and exhausted. But mostly I felt profoundly changed. I was convinced that there must be a reason for my cancer, and that I needed to address the way I live, not only to beat it but to fortify my body for life.

Now I've long advocated bodywork, meditation, and the benefits of Eastern medicine, so in addition to my Western treatment of a lumpectomy and six weeks of radiation, I had regular acupuncture and drank the "stinky teas" from the Tao of Wellness in Santa Monica. But my most life-changing discovery came two weeks after I was diagnosed, when my oncologist introduced me to Rachel, who surprised me with something I had never really thought about: What you eat matters immensely. And what I had been eating couldn't have been more wrong.

As I mentioned, I was very fit when I was diagnosed—I had just biked up Alpe d'Huez, one of the most famous climbs in the world. But since I had this impression of myself as healthy and invulnerable, I ate like a forty-year-old on the go, with most of my meals coming from hotel menus. That meant lots of pasta, club sandwiches, French fries, and Diet Coke. I didn't think that what I ate had any effect other than feeding my hunger and keeping me going.

Then I met Rachel, just before beginning my course of radiation. The sight was unforgettable: She walked into my house with a big bag of food and an even bigger bag of information that would forever transform the way I looked at what I put into my body. She taught me the inside story of nutrition, food by food, brand by brand, one tip and trick at a time. Rachel stressed the importance of antioxidants, omega-3s, high-fiber food, cancer-fighting components in spices, and eating seasonally and organically. Her ideas were all new to me. Even more important, her upbeat energy was contagious. For the first time, I felt empowered, as if I could now take a proactive stance in beating my breast cancer—and in fighting its return.

Rachel and I met frequently, and each time she taught me something eye-opening about how to eat defensively. At the same time, she didn't teach me anything crazy or extreme that would be hard to remember or follow. Everything made sense and seemed so easy. In fact, what makes Rachel's words really sink in aren't just the great ideas or her expertise—it's the way she delivers her advice. She doesn't lecture or go on and on about chemistry and biology. Instead, Rachel is all about getting real—we all live busy lives, so she keeps things easy, gets you into action doing what works, and teaches you not to wait to start living and feeling better. Even with her science and research background, she keeps it interesting and fun. That's what really made me want to share this amazing knowledge with all my friends. In fact, one of the first things I did after meeting Rachel was organize a party so she could inspire all my friends the way she inspired me. Just as I predicted, they loved hearing from Rachel as much as I did—and as I still do.

That's why I'm happy to see Rachel's expertise featured in this book. It's not just for cancer survivors—it's for everyone who wants to look better and feel better. It contains surprising info that even a busy person like me can use every single day, whether I'm hanging out at home or on the road. I bet you'll enjoy it too, and feel thoroughly empowered to take charge of your life. Even now, I can still hear Rachel's upbeat voice, saying, "Sheryl, this is your winning formula!" It really is.

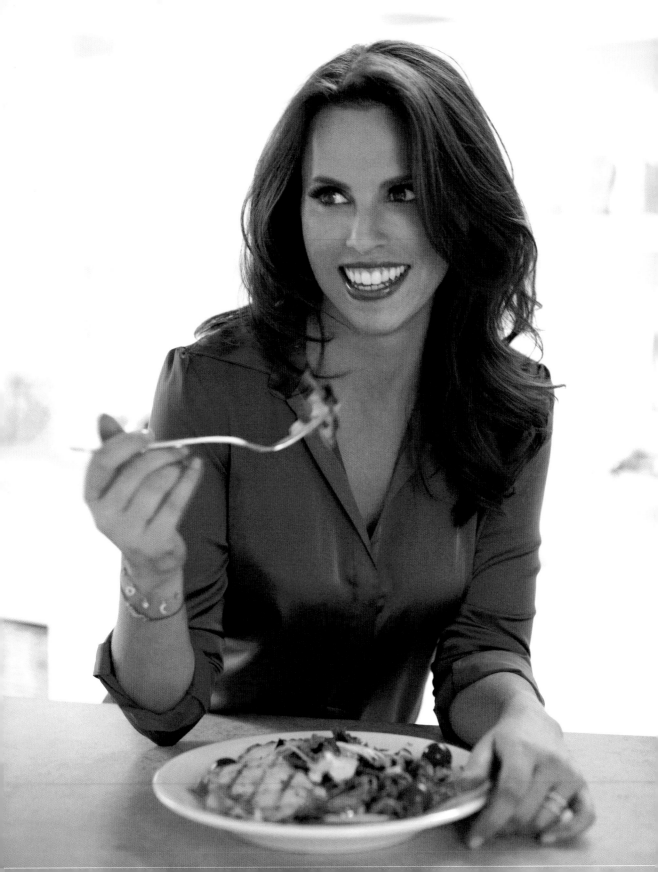

introduction
....

welcome to
eat to lose, eat to win

Ready to get skinny and healthy now? You've come to the right place!

The book you're reading right now is *not* your traditional diet book. The world doesn't need another dry, boring book about broccoli! What you do have is a realistic, cut-to-the-chase guide that translates nutrition and weight-loss science into your shopping cart. *In minutes, you can be on your way to the market.* You'll know what to get and how to put it all together so the pounds come off and the health benefits come on.

Patients tell me every day that they know what to do to lose weight. You probably do too! But it's not about knowing—it's about *doing.* So I'm cutting out all the stuff that could trip you up—the long lectures on weight loss and healthy eating, the confusing nutrition science, the complicated "phases"—and giving you just what you need to know to *leap right into action mode!*

Yes, I can make you thinner so you look better in a three-way mirror. That's the easy part! My real goal, however, is the synergistic effect of getting you thin *and* healthy. For life.

As a preventative nutrition researcher at medical centers, I've learned what works on both fronts. And it didn't include unnatural diets or food deprivation schemes. I started the Beller Nutritional Institute in Beverly Hills to give patients real, no-bull plans based on *science.* To help them understand and stick to those plans, I also provide lots of fun, easy-to-use tools they can get at a glance—from my trademark Food Autopsy™ analyses to visual shopping guides, all featuring pages and pages of photos. (Of food! What could be better?)

It's an approach that's helped Hollywood celebs, *Biggest Loser* and other reality show contestants, corporate execs, small-town homemakers, respected doctors, and countless others finally realize a winning formula they can own for life!

You are next.

All this ready-to-use-*now* advice I'll give you is dished out in four parts that go hand in hand:

Part 1 begins with jaw-dropping details on so-called healthy meals, which I call Food Autopsy analyses. (Sound scary? They are!) Then I'll show you how to build your breakfast, lunch, dinner, and snacks to help you look your best while never feeling like you're *ugh . . . on a diet.* My bottom line is to make the weight-loss process so simple that *you can't fail*!

In Part 2, I put it all together and outfit skinnylicious breakfasts, lunches, and dinners that are not only easy to assemble but good for you.

In Part 3, we go shopping! You'll see "buy this!" images of exactly what you should grab off the shelf. I've done the legwork for you, so you don't have to scour labels or memorize lists of "approved" foods. And rest assured: I have *no* ties to food companies, which means my recommendations come completely unbiased. I've simply translated complex nutritional science into simple tips to fill your shopping cart.

For sci-curious readers who want a more in-depth look at *why,* Part 4 offers the science behind the advice I'm giving you. I've deliberately kept the plan itself short and sweet so you can get started right away, but the research girl in me can never pass up the chance to help you learn a little something.

Hungry to get started? Then flip the page—it's time to *Eat to Lose, Eat to Win*!

rachel's action plan

FOR LOSING POUNDS AND WINNING PREVENTION

cutting to the truth: food autopsy™ alerts

Brace yourself! It's time for some
Food Autopsy analyses—a look inside
what's standing between you and skinny.

Scalpel . . . *Check*!

Magnifying glass . . . *Check*!

Now let's see what's *really* in that meal!

Sure, you know that a cheeseburger, fries, and a soda aren't exactly a slimming meal. You don't need a degree in nutrition to figure that out! In fact, *everyone* knows the basic formula for weight loss: Consume fewer calories than you burn. Simple, right?

Then why do so many people need help with it? Because what they *know* is often *wrong*. When you put many "light" and "healthy" foods under a nutritional magnifying glass, you see that they deliver a lot of diet-busting ingredients. And half the time people don't even know what hit them!

That's where I come in. My degree might say R.D., but I also play the role of dietary forensic specialist, dissecting and examining meals so the real truth comes out. I call them Food Autopsy analyses, and they've helped numerous patients slice through the hype of restaurant menus, frozen meals, and "innocent" salads to get their diets back on track.

The first time I ever did a Food Autopsy analysis, I was a researcher at Cedars-Sinai Medical Center in Los Angeles. Some of the doctors asked me to spot-check their lunches—and when I told them they were downing tons of calories and empty carbs disguised as healthy foods, they looked as if I had knocked the trays right out of their hands! I was *shocked* that I had shocked them. The food facts seemed so obvious.

That was my defining moment—and I've been doing Food Autopsy analyses ever since.

The Producer's Meal Doesn't Make the Cut

Fast-forward years later to the set of a popular TV series. The producer on the show was a woman obsessed with numbers—essential in an industry where budgets and ratings rule. And watching numbers is essential with diets too, right?

Unfortunately, her obsession with numbers—specifically, calories—led to a freezer stuffed with diet meals, all shouting "healthy" and "lean" and "lite"! Sure, the calories were low, but the producer hadn't read the entire script: ingredient lists that looked like a chem lab blew up in a salt mine. And none of these wannabe meals contained even one serving of filling vegetables. Without the satisfying volume, she wound up ordering one of those iced-blended diet killers whenever someone did a coffee run.

The bottom line: It doesn't matter whether you have an M.D. or an Emmy—when it comes to "healthy" meals, it's easy to develop a total disconnect between perception and reality.

That's why I'm kicking off this book with a few Food Autopsy analyses of some popular "good for you" dishes. You'll see eye-popping pictures of the calorie, carb, and sugar equivalents that are really lurking in there. (Keep in mind, these aren't always *nutritional equivalents*—we'll go into nutrition in later chapters.) I'm not against carbs and calories, by the way! If you're trying to lose weight, you need both in smart quantities. But if you're committing one of these fattening faux pas, that scale needle will never move down for you.

Don't worry, though! I'll also show you how to fix any mistakes so that bathroom gadget *will* finally listen.

The Top 6 "Healthy" Diet Mistakes

So shocking you'll never commit them again!

The frozen diet meal fanatic

Okay, let's look at that TV producer's lunch. The photo on the box looked like something from a French bistro. But once I popped it open, the packaging looked more substantial than the actual food inside. The bigger problem?

In this particular meal, the chicken is breaded, so it's basically a tiny piece of dark meat between two slices of white bread with some pasta on the side—the carb equivalent of three slices of bread. Throw in a sprinkle of veg for decor (one-eighth of a vegetable serving—no antioxidants or fiber for you!) and some sweet-and-salty mystery sauce and you've got a no-value meal.

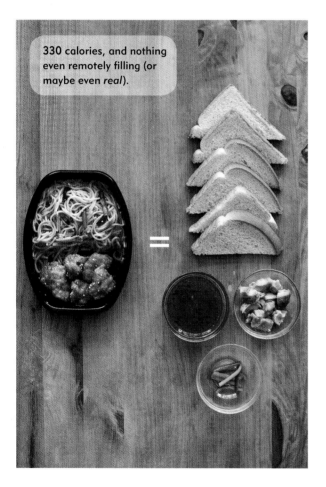

330 calories, and nothing even remotely filling (or maybe even *real*).

MY SOLUTION: When it comes to "lite" entrees, both quantity and quality matter! So forget those prepackaged, overprocessed excuses for meals. How about a frozen turkey (or salmon) burger warmed up and tossed over some bagged mixed greens with cucumber, a handful of cherry tomatoes, and a light dressing? Check out how great frozen *can* be.

320 calories and no preservatives!
Plus loads of healthy, sustaining veggies.

Sushi lovers—
get your carb OD right here!

Here's a typical—*typical!*—mistake. Some officemates escape for a "light lunch"—and wander into the most dangerous part of the neighborhood: the mall food court. There they find sushi. Perfect! Nothing deep-fried, no gravy or buttery sauces, lots of fresh ingredients. What's not to love? So they each order two rolls: a California roll and a spicy tuna roll. Well, let's see what they're really eating . . .

After consulting with sushi chefs and doing some nutritional digging, I got the inside scoop: A typical roll contains 290 to 350 calories and has the carb equivalent of 2½ to 4 slices of bread. So that California roll equals two sandwiches filled with imitation crab (processed fish), avocado, and a tiny bit of veg! Add the spicy tuna roll, and you're eating an additional 1½ tuna sandwiches with full-fat mayo. The message here: If you're trying to lose weight, "going on a roll" is not your best option!

MY SOLUTION: Not all sushi is bad—in fact, Japanese restaurants have many great options. The secret lies in *how* you order. First, request brown rice instead of white. With cut rolls, ask for "easy on the rice"—or, better yet, get hand rolls and "hold the rice." (You can request this even at the sushi counter at the grocery store.) Then add a side salad. That's the difference between a "light lunch" and a "right lunch."

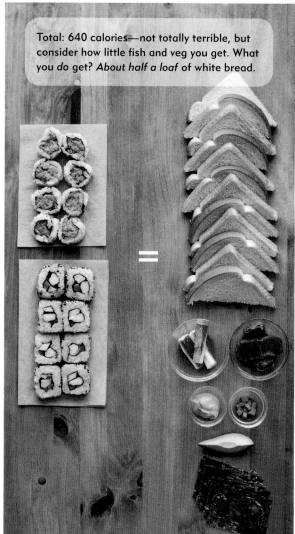

Total: 640 calories—not totally terrible, but consider how little fish and veg you get. What you do get? *About half a loaf* of white bread.

Now this is how we roll:
a combo of light rice and no rice.

The "I'll just have a salad" eater
(You won't believe what's hiding in there!)

One of my *Biggest Loser* contestants went to a popular chain restaurant and ordered her favorite salad: the usual lettuce with chicken and crunchy bits, like walnuts. The way she saw it, walnuts are good for you—they're rich in omega-3s.

But when I saw that salad, "omega-3" became "OMG."

Here's what the Food Autopsy analysis revealed:

Among those leafy greens hid a ton of sneaky ingredients: A thick vinaigrette, dried cranberries, and let's not forget the walnuts—make that *candied* walnuts. While these guys are healthy, they're hefty on calories. To top it all off, a total blanket of blue cheese. So if you're looking at the salad menu in search of skinny-health options, be warned: Many are way worse than the entrees!

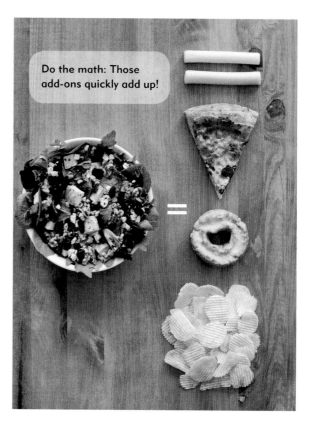

Do the math: Those add-ons quickly add up!

Typical Salad Add-Ons	Typical Amounts	Calories	Caloric Equivalent
Blue cheese	⅓ cup	160	2 string cheeses
Balsamic vinaigrette	4 tablespoons	200–320	1 slice of pizza
Candied walnuts	¼ cup	200	Glazed donut
Dried cranberries	¼ cup	130	Snack bag of potato chips

MY SOLUTION: Go for a heavy-on-the-greens salad with lots of colorful veg—then add a lean protein and a touch of fat (the dressing). For added crunch or a punch of flavor, look for salads with water chestnuts, snap peas, beets, hearts of palm, or oil-free sun-dried tomatoes. Craving cheese? Stay in caloric control by ordering it on the side and just adding a pinch. That's how you win on the scale: Keep it simple!

Now here's how you build a salad
(not an entire buffet in a bowl)!

Wrap your head around this major "DUI"

You can't miss 'em: Wraps are everywhere as a healthy lunch option—usually with the words "fresh" and even "natural" and "organic" applied to the ingredients. A friend of mine confidently picked one up at the grocery store as a "better" alternative to their sandwiches and burritos. And the next thing she knew, she was guilty of a DUI: Dining Under the Illusion (*it's good for me and my waistline too!*).

Well, I had to intervene. Food Autopsy time!

Here's the illusion: She thought she was getting her spinach fix—plus, that thin little wrap had to have fewer calories than two pieces of bread, didn't it? Think again. Less than 2 percent of the tortilla consisted of spinach *powder*. Aside from that, it was essentially colored white bread (courtesy of yellow #5 and blue #1) mixed with artificial flavors. What's more, the tortilla equaled nearly three times the calories and carbs of a slice of bread! And that's before I even looked at what was actually inside that wrap.

I had to reveal the hard news about her "fresh" lunch. After all, friends don't let friends DUI!

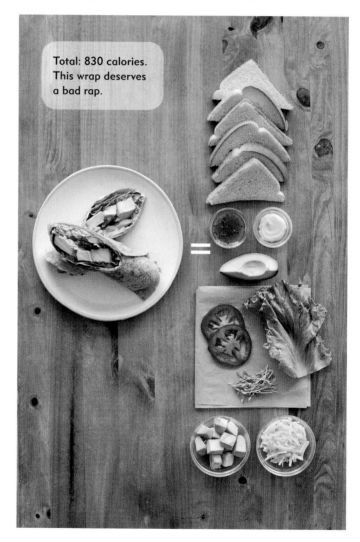

Total: 830 calories. This wrap deserves a bad rap.

MY SOLUTION: Ditch the three slices of colored white bread and score a value-full plate of real greens and tomato slices topped with grilled chicken. Dress it with avocado and add one slice of whole grain toast to make an open-faced sandwich. (An easy request at the deli.)

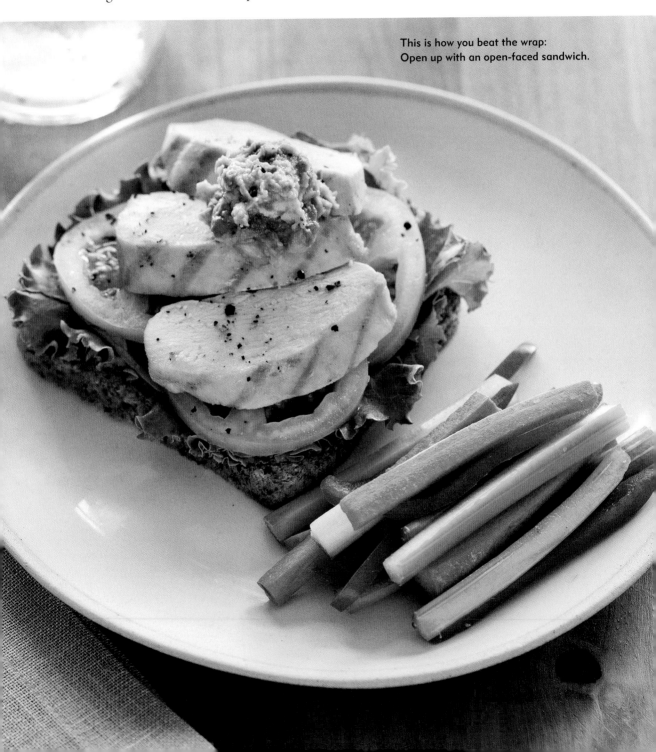

This is how you beat the wrap:
Open up with an open-faced sandwich.

The calorie *sipper* strikes again . . . and again . . . and again . . .

Every day in LA, I see people walking and driving around with their dietary problems in one hand. No, not donuts or sugar-bomb sodas—everyone knows those are lethal. I'm talking about the cup of steaming latte or organic juice they're confidently sipping away on.

Remember this: Just because you're not chewing it doesn't mean it's not costing you.

I told that to one of my patients who couldn't figure out why he wasn't losing weight. He told me he was following all my guidelines when it came to food, but then he confessed his beverages: Every day he started with a large vanilla soy latte—healthier than the mocha kind, right? Lunch included an organic lemonade from the health food store to go with a salad. And his late-afternoon pickup consisted of a green-tea energy drink.

None of that sounds bad, does it? Let's dive in:

TOTAL: 700 calories *just* in beverages, plus a jitter-inducing 141 grams of sugar— that's like eating 37 little lollipops in one day! (3.8 grams of sugar per lollipop.)

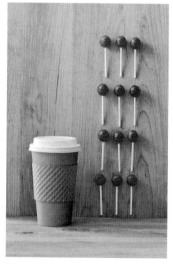

20-ounce vanilla soy latte

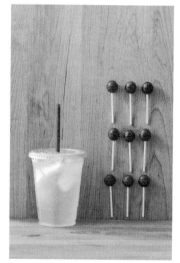

12-ounce glass of organic lemonade

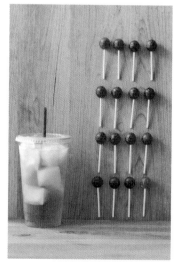

20-ounce bottle of green tea energy drink

MY SOLUTION: Train your palate not to crave intense sweetness—and save yourself all those diet-wrecking empty calories. Water is *always* the way to go. And you can punch up plain old H_2O in so many ways: Add a few frozen blueberries, slices of lemon, lime, orange, or cucumber, pomegranate seeds, or a few mint leaves. You can also go for an unsweetened iced or hot tea (my favorites are black or green matcha). For special occasions, make a "mocktail" by adding a tiny splash of pomegranate juice and a lime wedge to sparkling water. Yes, you can refresh without the excess!

No added sugars! I'll drink to that!

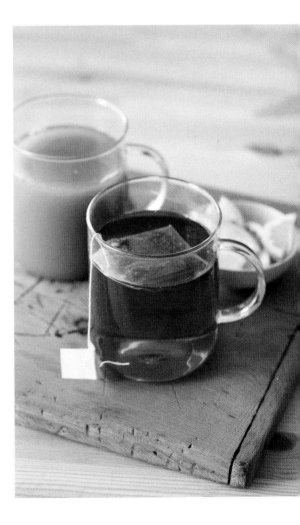

Vegan overkill!

I serve on the advisory boards of several health and medical organizations, so I couldn't believe what I saw at one of their annual meetings. We were all excited to dip into our catered vegan lunch, which promised "no refined sugars" on top of being completely meat- and dairy-free.

Then I did a double take at what looked like a double meal: On the plate was a portobello vegan tempeh burger slathered with vegan mayo and pesto sauce, plus a mound of kale salad tossed (more like doused) in a peanut sauce.

Kale is fantastic for you, and so are portobello mushrooms. And if you can replace animal proteins with vegetable-based ones in your diet, I'm all for it! But vegan doesn't mean "go all out!"

While everyone chowed down, I opted to have mine packed to go. I took this vegan specimen back to my lab for an extra-special autopsy.

What I found was that this one lunch packed approximately 1150 calories.

That's the caloric equivalent of a four-piece fried chicken meal with French fries on the side! Yes, the vegan-meal ingredients are healthier, but meatless doesn't always mean guiltless. Even healthy calories add pounds, and the caloric price tag on this meal will cost you.

So I was wrong: Add the sandwich and the salad together, and that wasn't a double meal—it was almost a *triple* meal. Going vegan is great, but eating three meals of anything in one sitting will send you up three pant sizes guaranteed, no matter what's on the plate.

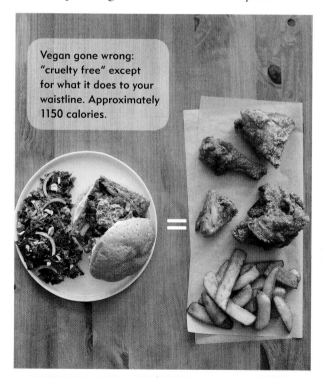

Vegan gone wrong: "cruelty free" except for what it does to your waistline. Approximately 1150 calories.

MY SOLUTION: Get all the flavor, and none of the guilt, with my vegan patty-and-mushroom open-faced sandwich and a side of kale. It's easy: Just take half a whole wheat bun and place a grilled tempeh patty on it. Add some grilled portobello slices and a spoonful of pomodoro sauce (like marinara sauce, only thicker). For your side, go with 1 cup of steamed kale with some diced tomato and lemon. And there you've gone vegan with total satisfaction, all at around 400 calories!

Remember that there's vegan and there's vegan done *right*. Regardless of what something is called—"vegan," "organic," "all-natural," "gluten-free," or "fresh"—you cannot overlook the supersized bun or the fact that it may be swimming in sauces and spreads. The fundamentals of healthy eating remain the same.

And that's where we start with the very next chapter.

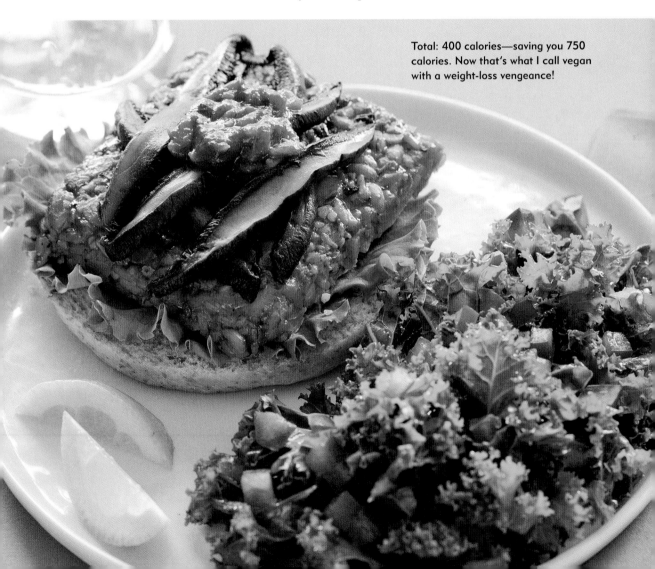

Total: 400 calories—saving you 750 calories. Now that's what I call vegan with a weight-loss vengeance!

get your a.m. fiber fix!

My favorite f-word—and why you need it first thing every day

You and I can't talk weight loss or better health without the f-word—and yes, I'm talking about fiber. I know, just hearing that word makes you think, *Oh, @*#$! Not another fiber lecture!*

And I agree. Fiber isn't sexy—I mean, who fantasizes about bran cakes? But hang in there, because I'm going to let you in on some info that I bet you've never heard about before—and that by the end of this chapter you'll have embraced it with both arms and a spoon. I've seen it happen so many times.

Need some motivation? Here's a true Hollywood story for you.

Getting Lucky in Hollywood

One of my patients is an A-list actress who always looks great, but she came to me intent on losing "those last seven pounds." (For Hollywood people, it's always *seven,* never the last five, like it is for everyone else. Maybe it's for luck?)

Anyway, despite working out with her personal trainer five days a week, she'd had *zero* luck losing even two pounds. Not surprising. Only some weight loss comes from exercise; the rest is all about your diet.

So I asked her what she usually eats for breakfast, and she gave me an answer I hear all the time: "I'm always on the run, don't have time to even think in the morning, and I wouldn't want a big meal anyway." So what does our shooting star eat for breakfast? A protein bar on her way out the door. Hey, her trainer had recommended it—it had to be good.

No. It wasn't.

When I performed a Food Autopsy analysis on that bar, I was horrified to find the wrong fats, various sugars, and a mere 3 grams of fiber amid 290 calories (a lot for such a teeny little thing). And it was processed to the max. I told her she had basically been eating a candy bar every morning. She turned white—absolutely mortified. "I've been eating *candy* for breakfast?! No wonder I've been crashing after an hour!" Now she was worried about her health too—not just her weight.

Fortunately, I had an easy fix for her problem: Ditch the bar and get that diet back on track by getting a lot more fiber at breakfast—all in a way that takes seconds to throw together and is totally tasty. A few weeks later? She was flaunting the results. All the pounds had dropped off, she had more energy, she wasn't ravenous an hour after breakfast, and she felt better too. She had joined my long list of fiber converts.

Now it's your turn!

4 Simple Rules to Make Fiber Work for *You*

I promise, there's nothing rocket science-y about this. Get the basic rules down, get started, and the whole eat-more-fiber thing will quickly become second nature. It will also help make your most important meal of the day (breakfast!) completely foolproof—so you'll lose weight without even having to think about it, *and* give your health a big boost.

RULE #1: You need 30 to 35 grams of fiber every single day. Lock that into your memory bank!

This is the magic number women should shoot for. Refer to it as your Daily 35. (For men, it's 35 to 40 grams.) And there are so many weight-related reasons to do it. For starters, high-fiber meals lengthen the presence of a hormone that sends the "I'm full!" signal to the brain—so you'll naturally put your fork down sooner and be far less likely to overeat. Fiber is also filling. It kind of puffs up in your system, which in turn helps you feel satisfied faster. Plus, high-fiber foods tend to be lower in calories and more diet-friendly in the first place.

WHAT *IS* FIBER, ANYWAY—AND WHAT DOES IT DO FOR ME?

It's not about what fiber does; it's all about what fiber takes *away*. You know that spa feeling: refreshed, tingly, *cleaned?* Well, your insides want that action too—every single day. And fiber has the marvelous ability to grab excess hormones like estrogen, cholesterol, and other potentially harmful compounds and whisk them out of the body. It's ridding you of toxins that, if left to linger too long in your digestive tract, could cause damage, including upping your risk of breast and colon cancer, as well as other diseases (see Part 4 if you want the full-on science). Not only does fiber make you feel satisfied and prevent overeating, it also delivers your daily dose of detox. So forget those quick-fix diet fads *du jour*, which are questionable and possibly hazardous. To look and feel your best—not just for a day but for life—you need to get your fiber on.

There are two types of fiber—soluble and insoluble—which work together like an internal spa team.

- Insoluble fiber acts like an exfoliant, gently scrubbing your digestive tract. (Imagine a microscopic loofah.)

- Soluble fiber works like a sponge, soaking up any icky stuff that's been sloughed off and ferrying it out of your body.

Don't worry about how much of what type you're getting. Too confusing! Just know that you need both—and they usually come as a package deal anyway.

Another major bonus: Some research suggests that fiber actually blocks the absorption of some of the calories in the foods you eat. Think of it as nature's version of a fat-blocking diet pill.

Getting 30 to 35 grams may seem doable at first glance, but the fact is that most of us aren't consuming even *half* this amount. Indeed, stats show that the average American gets a measly 11 to 15 grams a day—and that's on their "good days." But you don't have to be the average American. You're going to be above average!

RULE #2: Vegging out ain't enough!

You could inhale salad until you turned chlorophyll green and you'd barely get 15 grams before midnight. When I tell my patients this, I can hear their jaws hit the floor. Yes, you still must eat your fruits and veg (nice try!)—there's a lot more value to them than just fiber. But unless you eat a path through a small forest or farm, you won't get close to your Daily 35. Take a look at how the fiber numbers add up (or, rather, don't) over the course of the day:

TOTAL FIBER: 24 grams. *11 grams* **short of your Daily 35!**

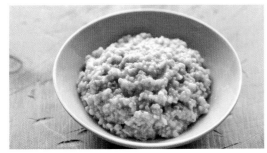

Breakfast: Oatmeal—4 grams fiber

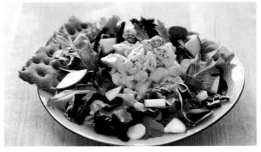

Lunch: Egg Salad and Cracker—6 grams fiber

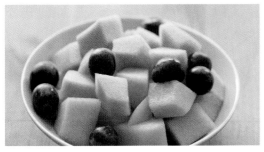

Snack: Fruit Bowl— 5 grams fiber

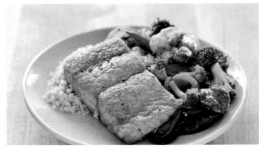

Dinner: Fish n' Veg—9 grams fiber

FRUSTRATING FIBER STATS

Wait, that's it?! Here's how much fiber various fruits and vegetables *really* contain per serving (in grams).

Banana, 1 medium	2.8	Carrots, ½ cup, cooked	2.3
Apple (with skin), 1 medium	4.3	Broccoli, ½ cup, cooked	2.5
Pear (with skin), 1 medium	4.0	Zucchini, ½ cup, cooked	0.9
Raspberries, ½ cup	4.0	Tomato, 1 small, raw	1.5
Blueberries, ½ cup	1.7	Cauliflower, ½ cup, cooked	1.4
Peach (with skin), 1 medium	2.2	Asparagus, ½ cup, cooked	1.8
Cantaloupe, ¼ melon	1.2	Lettuce, 1 cup, raw	0.9
Grapes, 20	0.9	Mushrooms, ½ cup, raw	0.5
Watermelon, 1 cup	0.6	Cucumber, ½ cup, raw	0.4

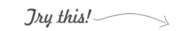 *Try this!*

MY TRICK OF THE TRADE "GASOLUTION"

If you fiber overachieve one day and need a little, um, relief, put a teaspoon of fennel seeds (in the spice aisle of any market) in a tea ball and steep into chamomile or other herbal tea for 2 to 3 minutes. Relieves excess gas like *that*.

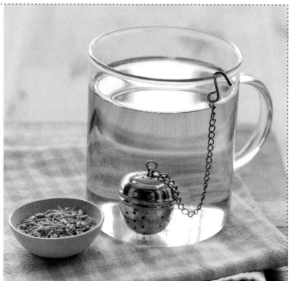

RULE #3: Not all fiber is created equal—go for the real deal!

I've met a lot of amazingly creative "industry people" in Hollywood, but the award for making up stories—and getting people to believe them—goes to some food manufacturers. They slap all sorts of promising words on their labels. They want you so hooked on the hype on the front of the package that you won't flip it over and check out the real nutrition facts and ingredients—but that's exactly where you need to go first.

You know that "high fiber!" claim you read? It may be true, but what you often get are "isolated fibers," which are extracted from whole foods that are rich in fiber and then added to other foods to boost the label's fiber count. Although these manufactured fibers aren't harmful, there's some sketchiness as to whether they have the same health benefits as whole food sources of fiber. So try not to rely on them as a main source of your Daily 35. Here are a few forms of these manufactured fibers:

- Inulin (chicory root extract)
- Arabic, acacia, and guar gums
- Corn and tapioca starch fiber
- Maltodextrin
- Polydextrose
- Soy fiber
- Cellulose fiber
- Cottonseed fiber

If you see a bunch of them on the label, yell "*cut!*" and move on. Go for the real deal!

RULE #4: And . . . *action!* Start every day with 10 to 15 grams of fiber— it's your fiber insurance strategy.

If you're like me, you take a few minutes every morning to spruce yourself up: face, hair, shoes, clothes, accessories, then back to shoes. Now I want you to add just one more item to that routine: a high-fiber breakfast containing at least 10 grams of your Daily 35.

Make this your new a.m. mantra: moisturize . . . accessorize . . . *fiberize.*

Why morning? 'Cause it's the easiest meal of the day to slip it in, as many of the highest-fiber foods tend to be cereals and grains that lend themselves to a.m. eating. And by loading up on fiber first thing, you won't have to count grams all day. Your most important meal will become a completely foolproof way to get to your 35-gram goal—and you'll lose weight and boost your health!

So don't waste your time on fat-bomb breakfast sandwiches or cereals consisting of air and sugar, or fake brown breads made with processed white flour and molasses for color.

Instead, use your morning meal to score your fiber insurance—which will also help stabilize your blood sugar before that lethal 10 a.m. status meeting. (It's not just coffee that keeps you alert during mind-numbing PowerPoint presentations!) Here are some smart ways to do just that.

What's for breakfast? Here are your fiber insurance guidelines:

Don't give yourself a migraine memorizing this stuff—I've already read the labels and done the legwork for you, so feel free to skip right to Part 3 and start shopping. These are just general good-to-know rules. Oh, and in all cases, try to go organic whenever possible.

Cereal

The Great Wall of Cereal may be the most intimidating section of the supermarket. With so many flavors and ingredients and health claims, no wonder most shoppers go with well-known brands or what's on sale! It's time to eliminate all that confusion. I'll tell you what to look for in a cereal:

- Per cup, your cereal should contain:
  - less than 200 calories
  - around 10 grams of fiber
  - no more than 10 grams of sugar

- Most of the fiber should be the real deal (from whole food sources), not isolated fibers.

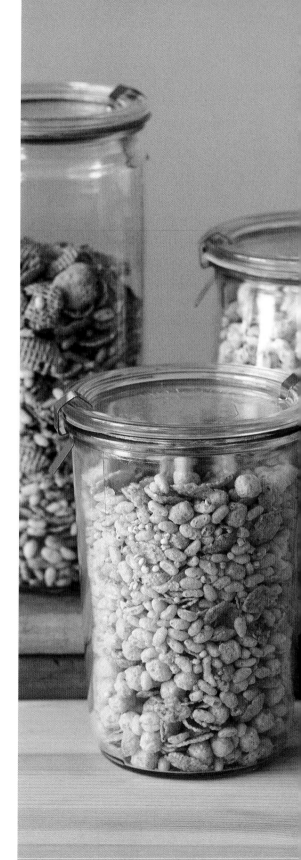

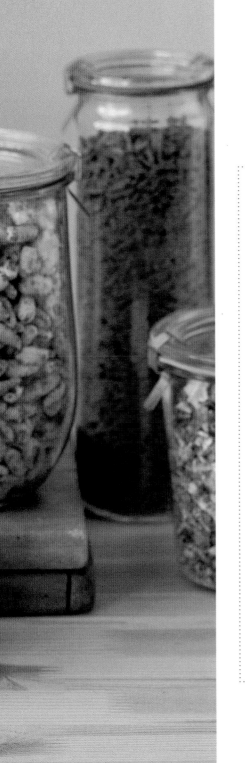

So many cereals =
so much confusion!

- Avoid cereals with artificial colors, sweeteners, and preservatives. Your body doesn't like—or need—that stuff.

- Watch out for portion trickery! Some food companies distort their labels with unrealistic serving sizes—some a teensy ¼ or ⅔ cup—so the calories look appealingly low. But you know you'll want more than that! Read labels and redo the math for 1 cup.

CEREAL WITH *WHAT?*

No discussion of cereal would be complete without milk, right? And you've got many options beyond regular milk.

- **MILK OPTIONS (1-CUP SERVING):** Now, I'm a dairy moderate. I don't rule out cow's milk completely, but since you have so many choices, I'd rather you experiment with something that wasn't squeezed from an animal. My personal favorites are almond, soy, hemp, coconut, and rice milk. Just look for unsweetened or light varieties fortified with calcium and vitamin D. If you just can't do without cow's milk, choose organic skim, which contains no added hormones and no unhealthy saturated fat.

- **NONFAT GREEK YOGURT (6-OUNCE SERVING):** Regular nonfat yogurt is okay, but the Greek kind dishes out way more protein, which will keep you satisfied and energized long after the cereal carbs burn off. Plus, most yogurts, including Greek, contain immunity-enhancing probiotics that also aid in digestive health.

Oatmeal

Cook up some steel-cut oatmeal, pour in almond or soy milk, add a dash of cinnamon and some sliced fruit and chia seeds or flaxseeds (I'll give you the scoop on those in a sec), and you've got one powerhouse of a meal. Just one bowl will fill your belly with warmth and provide steady energy until lunch. Best of all, you'll meet your a.m. fiber insurance goal with 12 grams—easy.

- Remember this oatmeal rule: The longer it takes to cook, the better it is for you. Steel-cut oats need 30 to 45 minutes, but they're also a superstar whole grain that's chewier and takes longer to digest. That means stable blood sugar levels all morning—no crashing. Quick-cooking steel-cut oatmeal comes in a nutritional second and can be prepped in 5 to 7 minutes. Rolled oats cook and digest faster, but are still a good, wholesome option. Got absolutely *no* time to cook? You can actually eat uncooked rolled oats with some fruit and cold milk (think cereal).

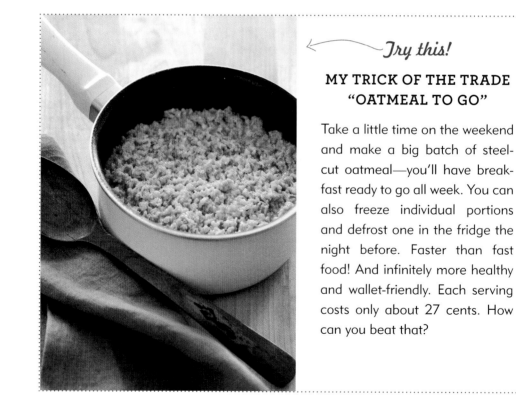

Try this!

MY TRICK OF THE TRADE "OATMEAL TO GO"

Take a little time on the weekend and make a big batch of steel-cut oatmeal—you'll have breakfast ready to go all week. You can also freeze individual portions and defrost one in the fridge the night before. Faster than fast food! And infinitely more healthy and wallet-friendly. Each serving costs only about 27 cents. How can you beat that?

FAB FIBER BOOSTERS

You know how a pair of cheap shoes won't take you the distance? Same with your typical breakfasts: You may need to add an extra dose of fiber to your oatmeal, cereal, or yogurt. The market offers a bewildering mess of fiber-boosting choices, so what should you look for? Here are my two top picks:

1. CHIA SEED. My ultimate favorite! It's got fiber, omega-3s, and lots of antioxidants. Tip: Be sure to get the *white* variety, because dark chia's charcoal color (shown at the top of this photo) makes it resemble what one of the *Biggest Loser* contestants jokingly dubbed "little bugs." Not so appetizing, and not something you'll stick with! Chia absorbs up to twelve times its own weight and expands your stomach—making it an amazing appetite curber. So adding a tablespoon of chia seeds to your diet can help you eat less, lower the number of calories your body absorbs from the foods you eat (the fiber effect), and double the amount of fiber you get. Love!

2. GROUND FLAXSEED. In addition to fiber, flaxseed offers omega-3s and lignans—a compound that may reduce the risk of breast and prostate cancers. It has an earthy, nutty flavor, and you need to grind it to score the full benefits. If you buy it ground, make sure it's vacuum-packed, then refrigerate in an airtight container. It will keep well for about forty-five to sixty days.

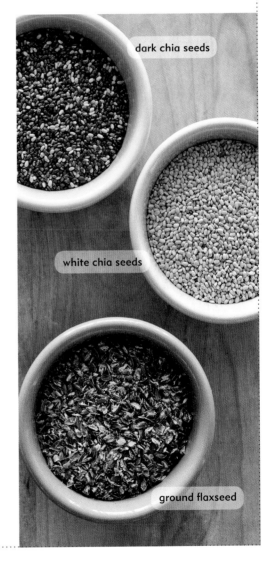

dark chia seeds

white chia seeds

ground flaxseed

- Portion wisely. Stick to ½ cup of rolled oats or 1 cup of cooked oats.

- Boost the fiber! With oatmeal, this is a *must*. Good as it is, oatmeal only contains about 4 grams of fiber per serving. So give it a double boost by adding a full serving of fruit such as apple, pear, or berries (around 4 grams) and one of my favorite seeds of choice (about another 4 grams). (See the Fab Fiber Boosters on page 27 for a list of seeds to try.) You'll meet your a.m. fiber insurance goal of 10 to 15 grams, no problem.

- Try to avoid instant oatmeal, as it not only digests faster but often contains added salt, sugar, and other ingredients to improve flavor, texture, and stability. Same with those flavored oatmeal packets, which may contain more undesirable ingredients than a tube of hot pink lipstick, plus tons of sugar, sodium, and unhealthy oils.

rachel's shaker-waker-upper

Here's a special mix to shake up your mornings and spice up your health with antioxidants. Just fill an empty spice shaker with an equal mix of:

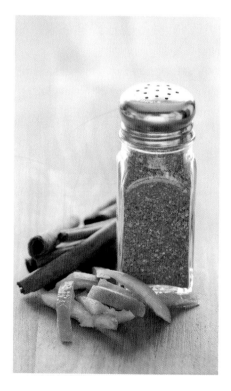

- Ceylon cinnamon

- Dried orange peel (found in the spice aisle of your local market, but watch out: peels are pesticide heavy, so go organic)

- Ground chia seeds (optional)

Why I love it:

- Cinnamon has tons of potential benefits, including weight loss, anti-nausea, and cholesterol reduction.

- Orange peel may suppress appetite and aid digestion (hello, weight loss!). It also contains D-limonene and hesperidin—anti-inflammatory enzymes that could help slow down aging and prevent cancer, *especially* breast cancer.

Sprinkle some Shaker-Waker-Upper on any high-fiber foods, such as whole grain French toast, cereal, or a bowl of raspberries or oatmeal. That'll give your breakfast a dash of get-up-and-go that's also good-to-go. (Later I'll introduce you to my Magical Mystery Mix—or MMM—for lunch and dinner.)

Bread—and other items from the massively confusing bread aisle

The bread section can be as head-spinning as the Great Wall of Cereal—with every wrapper shouting various promises, like "fiber rich!" and "wholesome goodness!" Uh-huh. *Not.* Here's how to find the good ones:

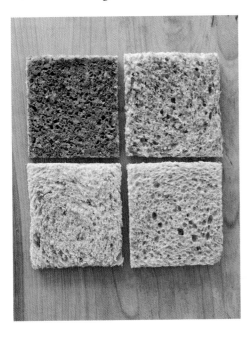

- Each slice (or tortilla, pita, whatever) should have:
    - at least 3 grams of real fiber
    - no more than 90 calories

- "Whole grain" or "whole wheat" should be the very first thing on the ingredients list. Some breads say "multi-grain" or "made with whole wheat," but what matters is the first ingredient. If the label says "enriched wheat flour," don't throw it in your cart—just see how far you can throw it, *period.*

- Avoid any bread that contains high-fructose corn syrup or artificial sweeteners.

GIVE BREAD THE SQUEEZE TEST!

Here's a quick trick to measure a bread's true value: Take a slice and, yes, squeeze it. If you can easily squish it into a marble-size ball, you're better off feeding that bread to the pigeons. Odds are it contains very little real fiber and consists mostly of empty carbs and isolated fibers (you might as well rip open a sugar packet and snort the contents).

My Squeeze Test is a much better health gauge than going by color, because many brown breads are simply white bread with a dash of added caramel or molasses to make them *appear* healthy. (Amazing that's legal!) A truly good bread will break or crumble when squeezed, since it contains whole or pieces of grains (not just whole grain flour).

Of course, if you do any serious squeezing in the supermarket, you might find yourself face to face with the security guard. So just give the bagged loaf a gentle press, which should still give you a good idea if it's a keeper. It should feel dense, not like a cheap hotel pillow.

The Squeeze Test works! (But not something to try in a supermarket. Trust me.)

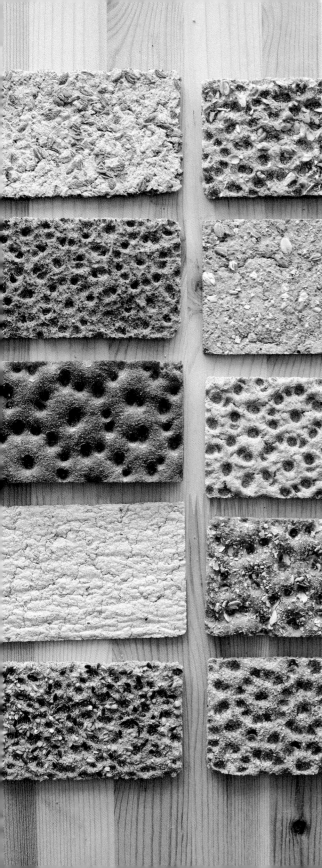

- Look for visible whole grains or pieces of whole grains within the slices—not just sprinkled on top of the loaf. This indicates that it's not just whole grain flour (and better for blood sugars).

- It needs to pass my Squeeze Test (see page 30).

Crackers

Crackers—for *breakfast*? Why not?! They've come a long way since the saltine. (Empty carbs and salt, anyone?) Indeed, crackers actually make a great bread substitute, since they require no toasting, deliver great crunch, and are extremely versatile. But choose carefully! Most are so hyper-refined they're almost *non*foods.

- Keep the calories around 70 to 90 per serving. For a meal like breakfast, a few servings is okay—so the calories wind up 150 to 200 total, similar to what you'd get with cereal.

- Go big! I've found that boxes filled with little pieces are too easy to snack on and on and on. Look for crackers that come in larger sheets—which also stand in better for bread and feel like a real meal rather than a nibble.

- Each large cracker should have at least 2 grams of fiber.

- Make sure the first ingredient listed on the back of the package is "whole grain," "whole wheat," or "whole rye."

- If you see high-fructose corn syrup or artificial ingredients on the label, put the box back on the shelf.

- Look for visible grains or seeds. They add both flavor and nutrition.

That's it! Simple rules and lots of choices for you.

Want some specific ideas about how to put together a complete breakfast? Check out the menu options in Part 2! I promise, you'll have this whole fiber thing dialed in no time—and reap the skinnifying health benefits.

YOUR FIBER CHEAT SHEET

- You need 30 to 35 grams of fiber per day—35 to 40 for guys. But start gradually.

- Fibersize your breakfast: Aim to get 10 to 15 grams of your daily total in the a.m.—it's your fiber insurance plan!

- Keep your breakfast under 350 calories when putting together an improv meal, but *never* forget your minimum fiber requirement. The breakfast suggestions here—and in Part 2—automatically do that for you, no tallying required. This guideline is just for when you need to DIY (at an airport, when you're out of town, or your market doesn't have the recommended items).

- Bonus points for boosting the fiber in your breakfast with white chia seeds or flaxseeds!

- Beware of manufactured fibers like inulin, maltodextrin, oat fiber, and cellulose fiber (although harmless, their value is questionable).

- Now all that's left for you to do is **go shopping**! Jump to Part 3 to get started!

WATCH OUT! HOW GRAB-AND-GO CAN TURN INTO A STUFF-AND-CRASH BREAKFAST

One of my patients is a college student trying to lose her freshman fifteen. I give her my standard breakfast talk about cereal with yogurt or oatmeal—and she quickly says that won't work. That's because her favorite can't-live-without-it invention is the snooze alarm, so she's behind schedule before her feet even hit the floor.

What does this girl on the go do for breakfast? Get ready for it: On the way to class every day, she stops by a coffee shop for a caffeine fix and a reduced-fat blueberry muffin. She's done the mental algebra: reduced fat = diet friendly; blueberries = fruit, right? Unfortunately, that "right" couldn't be more wrong. Time for a Food Autopsy snapshot!

Calorically, that muffin equals two glazed donuts with salt dumped on top. Seriously! The lesson here: Just because an item is "reduced fat" doesn't mean it's low in calories. This one tipped the scales at 410 calories (and only 2 grams of fiber) and packed in *10 teaspoons* worth of sugar! That's a recipe for a crash—no wonder she kept falling asleep in class. (Don't blame the professor!)

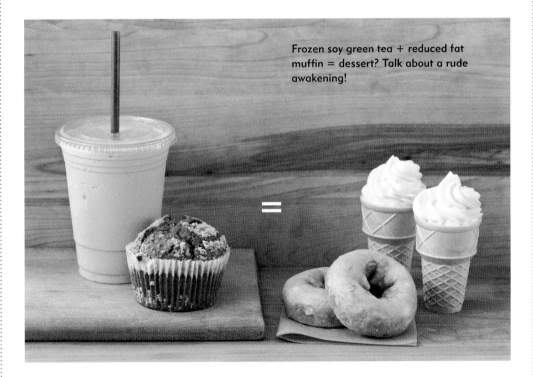

Frozen soy green tea + reduced fat muffin = dessert? Talk about a rude awakening!

As for her iced blended soy green tea? For all the magic words—"soy" and "green tea"—there's a reason it tastes like a shake. Because it *is* a shake! From a caloric standpoint, she might as well have eaten two small ice cream cones! Even without the whipped cream, it tacks on another 310 calories and 16 teaspoons of added sugar to her breakfast. Not to mention, it practically costs more than her student loans! This jeans-stretching, constipating, gas-forming concoction should be tossed to the curb.

The total for her grab-and-go? A whopping 720 calories and 26 teaspoons of sugar! Her freshman fifteen was on the fast track to becoming the freshman *thirty*.

So what's a girl on the go to do? Try one of these **fiber-sized grab-and-go breakfast options**! They changed my patient's life—and dress size! You're next.

SOLO CUP FILLED WITH CEREAL. Remember those big red plastic cups that got passed out at every frat party in college? Oh, yes, you do. Well, they happen to be the perfect size for a nutritious meal. Toss in 1 cup of your favorite high-fiber cereal, add your milk of choice, grab a plastic spoon, and hit the road. You can finish it (without spillage) while you're stuck in rush hour traffic or waiting for the bus. (Green tip: You can always wash and reuse the cup—or sub in a coffee mug.)

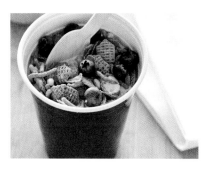

GNU FLAVOR & FIBER BAR CRUMBLED ON TOP OF 6 OUNCES OF NONFAT GREEK YOGURT. One of my favorite at-your-desk options! (See page 184.)

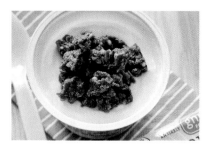

4 WASA CRACKERS, A WEDGE OF LAUGHING COW LIGHT CHEESE, A HARD-BOILED EGG, AND 2 CLEMENTINES. It doesn't get more portable than this! Stash everything in a little bag and snatch it on your way out the door.

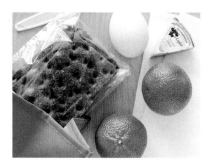

flip your meals—
and forget counting calories

My failproof strategy for skinny (but delish) lunches and dinners

Lights . . . camera . . . wait a sec!

So there I was, getting to know the *Biggest Loser* contestants before the season began. No way would I go in front of the cameras without knowing their eating habits first. I'd rather go on air without makeup. Well, almost.

At first I was pleasantly surprised: Most of the contestants had already made big-time healthy strides—eating less fast food, cooking more for themselves, and making better choices in general.

Then I actually saw one contestant's dinner: grilled chicken breast, whole wheat pasta with marinara sauce, pine nuts, and a touch of veg. OMG—I could barely look.

The Biggest Loser's Big Mistake

I know what you're thinking: Hold on, Rachel, what's wrong with that? The pasta's whole wheat! The sauce and pine nuts are healthy! That's lean protein! And there's veg on her plate, too!

Yes, you're right. Those are all good choices. The problem? The meal was completely backward!

I'm not saying she ate dessert first. I'm talking about the *priorities* on her plate. The chicken breast was the size of a brick—a brick on steroids. The mountain of pasta she'd dished out had practically collected snow at its peak. And the veg portion was so tiny, it was more after-thought than actual serving.

The result? Mega meal overload.

This poor contestant had committed the classic American mistake of making protein the center of her meal, then thinking carbs, and last (and certainly least!) adding a token amount of veg. When I revealed how many calories she really had on her plate (see Pasta Night Flip-aroni, page 37), her eyeballs practically popped out. That one mistake had negated all her weight-loss efforts.

She wasn't alone.

Most of the contestants had their meals backward. They needed a whole new way to look at eating—a way so simple and automatic, it would be a total no-brainer. Let me show you!

Rachel's Flip-It Method

Take whatever you think about meals and turn it completely upside down: Think *veggies first,* lean protein next, then a touch of healthy fat—and, last of all, a modest serving of complex carbs.

I know, it sounds totally un-American. Next thing you know, I'll be telling you to drive on the wrong side of the road. But if you use my Flip-It Method, you can't fail!

There's no counting calories. No weighing portions. No skipping what *matters.* You'll automatically get around 400 to 550 calories at lunch and dinner—*plus* loads of antioxidants, which are as important to your body as weight loss.

You want to know the best part? You get to really *eat.*

Take a look at how dramatically the Flip-It Method leaned out this Biggest Loser's plate, while still leaving lots to eat. Seeing is believing.

Okay, you may be saying, "Flipping pasta is easy! But how do you flip a burger? It looks the same either way—bun on top, bun on bottom . . ." As the fast food commercial goes, think outside the bun! Here's what another contestant did to save tons of calories at a burger joint.

He made healthier swaps—regular burger for a turkey burger, regular fries for sweet potato fries—but was it enough? Take a look at both the pre-flipped and post-flipped meals, and see what a BIG difference a flip can make!

PASTA NIGHT FLIPARONI:
HOW ONE CONTESTANT GOT HER PRIORITIES STRAIGHT

the pre-flipped pasta plate

2 cups cooked whole wheat pasta: *Waaay* heavy. That's nearly a full meal's worth of calories before adding anything else to the dish!

8 ounces grilled chicken breast: Did that chicken breast get an implant?

½ cup marinara sauce: Small calories, big health benefits from the tomatoes—now that's a keeper!

4 tablespoons grated Parmesan cheese: Big flavor in a dash, but much more than she needed.

¼ cup pine nuts: Nuts are great, but going nuts on nuts will cost you.

½ cup veg cooked in 2 teaspoons of oil: a measly ½ cup? Are we decorating here?

TOTAL CALORIES: 1221. *Mamma mia!* That's more than two dinners on one plate!

the flipped pasta plate

½ cup cooked whole wheat pasta: You still get your pasta fix *and* keep your waistline from becoming a coastline.

3 ounces grilled chicken breast: Now that's a more reasonable portion—and it still feels substantial.

½ cup marinara sauce: No skimping here. This delivers major flavor and antioxidant power (well hello, lycopene!). Warning: Watch the sugar and salt content in store-bought brands.

1 tablespoon grated Parmesan cheese: The perfect amount for a flavor punch—and for just 30 calories.

2 cups vegetables sautéed in a little olive oil: Ah, here comes the filling, good-for-you stuff! *This* should be your meal base—not the pasta. Multi veg = multi vitamins!

TOTAL CALORIES: 411. By flipping the meal she saved a whopping 810 calories, scored more antioxidants, and still got to savor a full pasta meal.

FLIPPIN' BURGERS:
BECAUSE YOU DON'T WANT TO SUPERSIZE *YOURSELF*

the pre-flipped burger

1 lettuce leaf, 1 tomato slice, and sliced pickles: If your veggies are so thin you can see through them, they don't count as a serving.

1 slice American cheese: Extra fat, extra processed! All packed in 1 tiny ounce.

1 tablespoon mayo: Yikes! (Enough said.)

1 to 2 teaspoons ketchup: Most restaurant ketchups = high-fructose corn syrup. Go easy!

1 hamburger bun: Want big buns? You'll get 'em with this typical hamburger holder. It's the carb equivalent of 3 slices of white bread!

Large order of sweet potato fries: At most places, they add more calories than the patty and bun together—just for a side!

4-ounce turkey burger patty: Typical restaurant serving.

TOTAL CALORIES: 1137. The number of years it will take to work this off!

the flipped burger

½ cup chopped tomato, cucumbers, carrots: The right way to fill up—do this for a few meals and you won't even know the fries are missing.

1 ounce feta cheese: Better flavor and less processed than American cheese.

1 tablespoon champagne vinegar and 2 teaspoons olive oil: A dash of healthy fat with some zing.

2 cups mixed greens: Because buns are so twentieth century. And it automatically keeps the waiter from asking, "You want fries with that?"

4-ounce turkey burger patty: You still get the burger!

TOTAL CALORIES: 390. You saved 747 calories. That's what I call a happy meal!

Inspired? Let's start flipping!

Here's your step-by-step guide to mastering the Flip-It Method at lunch and dinner.

STEP 1: Start every meal by flipping out with vegetables.

I swear, I'm not sentencing you to a life of salads. I'd lose my mind if that's all I ate too.

But if you want to lose weight *and* feel satisfied *and* get a dose of antioxidant protection, the strategy is so simple: veggies first. And except for starchy varieties (peas, corn, butternut squash, potatoes), *you can have as much as you like.* Seriously—veg out!

Do you have to go veggies-first 100 percent of the time? No. But aim for at least eleven meals out of your fourteen lunches and dinners in a week (it's okay to flex on the weekend a little). It's this easy:

- **HAVE A *MINIMUM* OF 1½ CUPS COOKED OR 2 CUPS RAW VEG PER MEAL**. That's much more than the transparent lettuce leaf and wafer-thin tomato slice you get in a typical sandwich. So if you're craving turkey on whole grain, have a pile of crunchy crudités on the side.

- **THINK BEYOND SALADS**. Yes, they're easy, but if you do 'em every day, you'll start planning unhealthy escapes. My view is: The only good dietary plans are *sustainable* ones. That means making meals you'll really want to eat. So in addition to salads, think bowls of gazpacho or chunky veg soup—they're just as good as a plate of vegetables. Roast some grape tomatoes in a little olive oil and balsamic vinegar and serve them warm next to a piece of grilled fish. Or grill veggie kabobs to go with skewers of shrimp.

- **USE THE FLIP-IT METHOD WHEN YOU EAT OUT, TOO**. You'll have to approach the menu differently—because unless you're at a vegan joint, no description of a dish ever starts with "sautéed fresh kale." It's always the protein that gets top billing. Here's what I do: Spot a veg you like on the menu and ask for your protein entree to be served with that veg. Easy on the oil, of course.

Notice I didn't say anything about steaming your vegetables? Nothing wrong with that—except it reminds me of my desperate dieting days, when I believed that the secret to shedding pounds was to bore my mouth to death. *Shudder.*

Fortunately, I discovered the cookie sheet. Easy there—I'm not talking snickerdoodles. We're still doing veggies first, but in an easy and deliciously awesome way. No joke! Ask any of the TV show contestants I work with about my cookie sheet tricks and they'll get a wistful look in their eyes . . .

grab a cookie sheet—roast up some veg!

Feel free to share this starter-kit recipe with your friends. In fact, I insist that you do!

1. Toss precut, bagged veggies (preferably organic) like green beans, cauliflower, and multicolored bell peppers and any other veg you like on a cookie sheet, spray with olive oil, and season to taste (check out my Magical Mystery Mix below).

2. Throw it in a preheated 375°F oven.

3. Go check Facebook while the veggies roast. (But don't scout out your ex—it'll only make you want to eat or drink something bad for you.)

In 20 to 30 minutes you'll have yummy caramelized veg. Got leftovers? Mix them with fresh greens to make the base of tomorrow's lunch.

magical mystery mix—my trick of the trade

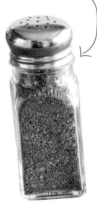

I call this the Magical Mystery Mix—because it's easy to remember, as it will make you go *MMM* . . . It not only adds a serious flavor kick to your roasted veggies, it's also loaded with anti-inflammatory and immunity-boosting ingredients and has absolutely zero calories. And it's so, so, *so* simple to make. Just take an empty salt shaker and fill it with roughly equal portions of:

- Turmeric
- Ground black pepper (go easier)
- Garlic powder
- Ground ginger (optional)

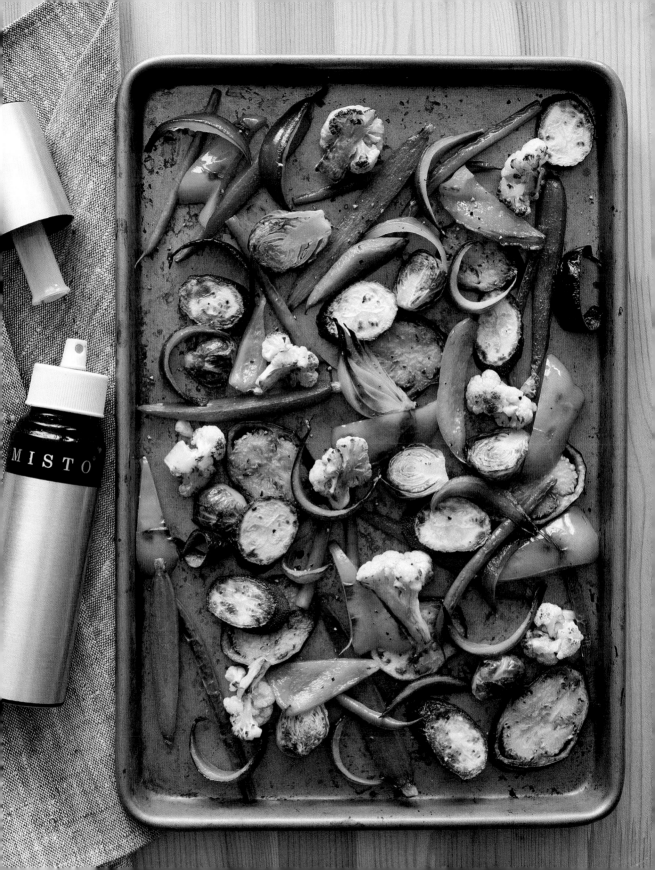

YOU GOTTA CRUISE TO LOSE

I don't care what you do with your social life, but when it comes to vegetables, I want you to date around. *With a vengeance.*

Go ahead, be a veggie slut.

Don't let your entire relationship with vegetables ride on your first impressions of spinach and broccoli. Spread the love. There are more kinds of veg showing up in the fresh food section every day, including some hot exotic numbers from halfway around the world, waiting for you to experiment with them.

Don't know how to prep them? Use that Internet you pay for every month. You'll literally find millions of recipes for everything from arugula to zucchini.

The hard-core full-frontal truth: If you want to lose weight and protect your body but refuse to eat your vegetables, you're going to be screwed. Your veg-less food portions will be so tiny that they'll leave you hungry and nutritionally deprived. You'll wind up eating more, and eating poorly—which will mean eating to gain, not to lose.

So cruise the produce section, pick two or three new things, and give 'em a shot! Play around with spices, sauces, soups, and salads. It's easier than you think. I've converted many reluctant veggie eaters in my career—and you're next on my list!

the right way to do fast food!

Got three minutes? That's all it takes to DIY and fly.

1. Toss handfuls of bagged precut greens into a portable container.

2. Top with some colorful precut bagged veggies.

3. Add a protein, such as one of your premade Sunday Salads (page 47) and an optional hard-boiled egg.

4. Stash in the fridge for the next day.

Now all you have to do is grab your DIY fast food on your way out the door to work. If you do that regularly, it will become as instinctive as grabbing your car keys. It's a winning solution to shedding pounds, and it's healthier and cheaper (about $3 for the whole thing) than ordering lunch. Best of all, you'll own the satisfaction of knowing your lunch is a done deal.

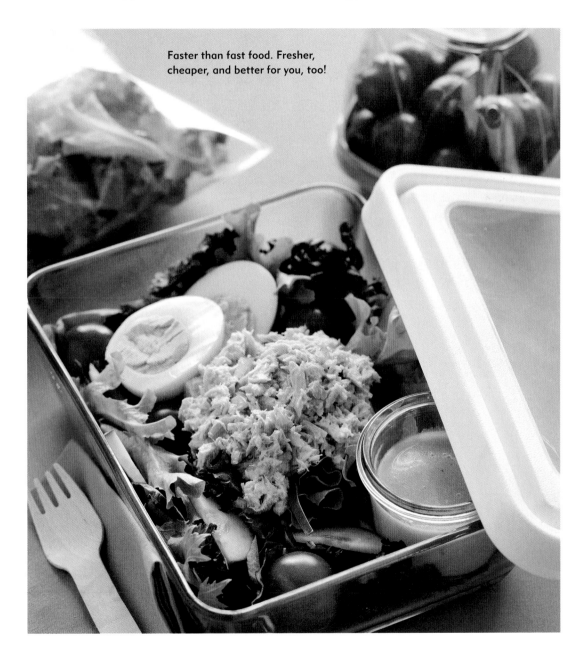

Faster than fast food. Fresher, cheaper, and better for you, too!

YOUR BACKUP PLAN: FROZEN ASSETS

If you can't handle fresh veggies—too expensive, too much work, too likely to go bad—then play it cool. Literally. Hit the frozen food section for your veg.

I know what you're thinking: *The freezer? For veggies?* You bet! They're picked at their peak and immediately frozen to lock in the nutrients. I'm not dissing fresh veggies, but many of them spend days or even weeks in transit, losing vitamins and minerals on the way (unless you buy from local farmers). Others are grown indoors, out of season and aren't as tasty. So believe it or not, frozen veg may offer more nutrition than the fresh stuff. They're also a good deal.

Plus, for those of us with hectic schedules (work, families, reality show contestants to consult and console), frozen veg are washed, peeled, and even prepped, which makes them the perfect backup. On those nights when you've got nothing in the fridge, don't call for Chinese takeout. Open the freezer instead. Grab a bag of stir-fry blend veggies (your meal base), add frozen chicken, shrimp, or a salmon burger, and you have a great meal.

How cool is that?

Sound Bite: Don't Add Snacks to Your Salad!

I love nuts and dried fruit, but they're calorically dense and *sooo* easy to overdo. Your no-brainer salad will get bloated with extra calories you can't afford if you want to lose weight. In fact, you'll essentially be eating lunch *and* your afternoon snack at the same time. If you really want them, add a *pinch*—not handfuls like most restaurants do. Smarter ways to add flavor and crunch to your salad: Toss in water chestnuts, snap peas, beets, hearts of palm, a few sliced olives, oil-free sun-dried tomatoes, or artichoke hearts. Oh, and you know that packet of crackers some restaurants give you with your salad? Pretend you didn't even see it.

STEP 2: Add some lean protein. (Lost between beef, beans, and everything in between? My Protein GPS will guide you!)

How to navigate through the world of proteins is one of the most common questions my patients ask. It's like being at the half-yearly sale at Nordstrom—they're excited by all the options but don't know where to start! Many find themselves stuck on the Big Three (that's chicken, turkey, and beef) for meal after meal after meal.

My solution? A system I call the Protein GPS.

Like that gadget in your car, the Protein GPS will help you find your way—but instead of streets and addresses, it will guide you through both plant- and animal-based proteins. And it's not something you plug in; it's a new way of thinking. The primary destination? A guiltless—yes, guiltless—solution for proteins.

Combined with the Flip-It Method, the Protein GPS won't steer you wrong. It works like this:

How to navigate proteins:

You have 7 lunches and 7 dinners each week—totaling 14 protein choices. Here's how you should dish them out:

- 4 meals with low-mercury, omega-3–rich fish (I'll make it easy!)
- 2 to 3 meals with beans
- 2 meals with tofu
- 2 to 3 meals with eggs
  TOTAL: 10 TO 12 MEALS

That leaves 2 to 4 meals open for the Big Three: lean chicken, turkey, or grass-fed beef (or any other lean protein you like). Except now they've become the *little three*—a much smaller part of your diet. By following the Protein GPS, you won't have much room for chicken, turkey, or beef by the end of the week—and you'll eat less by default. I'm not totally knocking these three. But research suggests that a diet emphasizing plant-based proteins is ideal for both weight and health. And if you're going to have animal proteins, why not go for ones with the most nutritional benefit? That's the whole idea behind my Protein GPS: to give you a good mix—one that's doable and doesn't require an extreme makeover.

Now let's dig in to my preferred protein choices—beginning with fish.

Get Hooked on Fish

Eat it: 4 times a week
A serving is: 3 to 4 ounces for women,
5 to 6 ounces for men (cooked)

Americans have no problem eating fish . . . as long as it's breaded, deep-fried beyond recognition, then drowned in tartar sauce. As you can probably guess, that's not the kind of fish serving I'm talking about.

Here's the big tasty plus—and why I put fish first on your Protein GPS: Done right, fish is a low-cal source of protein. And many kinds, such as wild salmon, trout, and black cod, are low in mercury *and* high in omega-3 fats, which can help reduce your risk for heart disease, certain cancers, and diabetes. Shrimp, crab, and scallops are slightly lower in omega-3s but are also great options. (For a longer list, see page 165.) It's skinny eating with a dose of prevention—totally my style!

HOW TO MAKE FISH FOUR TIMES A WEEK A REALITY

1. Order it in restaurants. This is the easiest option by far. But don't let the cook add butter or oils high in omega-6 fats (corn, soybean, vegetable)! This is so important that I have to repeat it: *Don't!* They cancel out the benefits from the omega-3s in your fish. A little olive oil is fine.

2. Quick-fix it once or twice at home. Don't panic—it's really, really easy. Much faster to prep than chicken, actually! Try my no-mess, five-minute trout with roasted tomatoes on page 135. It's a recipe I give to every new patient.

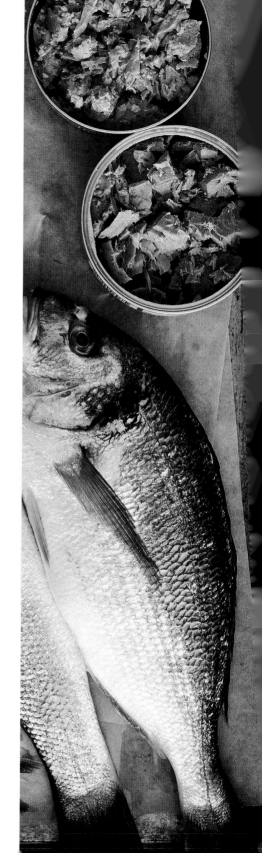

3. Tap into canned fish (your omega-3 insurance strategy!). One or two days a week, dive into a can of low-mercury wild tuna, salmon, or (gasp!) sardines. I'll give you a starter-kit recipe for some of these you can make on a lazy Sunday in minutes: My patients are so obsessed with how cheap and effortless this omega-3 fix is that they named it the Sunday Salad (even if they make it on a Wednesday). Make it once a week and you've guaranteed two of your four fish servings.

starter-kit recipe: sunday salad

Two 5- to 6-ounce cans low-mercury tuna or wild salmon
1 tablespoon reduced-fat Vegenaise (or substitute guacamole
    or Greek yogurt)
1 celery stalk, chopped, and/or ¼ cup chopped red onion or parsley

Mix all the ingredients in a bowl, drop a scoop on top of a fresh mixed-green salad, and voilà! The rest can live in the fridge for another two days.

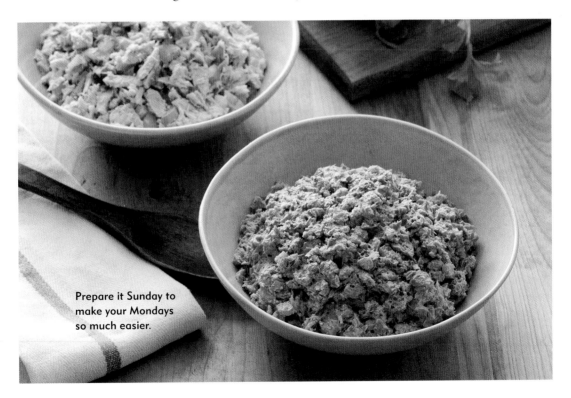

Prepare it Sunday to make your Mondays so much easier.

Let's Do Tofu!

Eat it: 2 times a week
A serving is: 6 to 8 ounces

I understand the hesitation. Most Americans think tofu is the punch line of a joke, or that soy is bad for them. It's not! In fact, research shows that tofu is *good* for you. It's also neutral tasting—all right, it's bland—but you can use that to your advantage and flavor it any way you like.

- First, buy straight-up firm traditional Asian tofu (sold in blocks) or tempeh (fermented soy). For about 20 cents extra, get the organic and sprouted varieties (non-GMO with more nutrition).

- Go super-easy on the wannabe meats, and be selective. You'll find all sorts of "sausage" patties and tofu hot dogs at the market, but they're generally expensive and overly processed (with soy concentrates and isolates).

So what do you do with all that tofu? (If I had a dollar for every time someone asked me that, I could buy a season's worth of Louboutins!) Here's my favorite easy recipe . . .

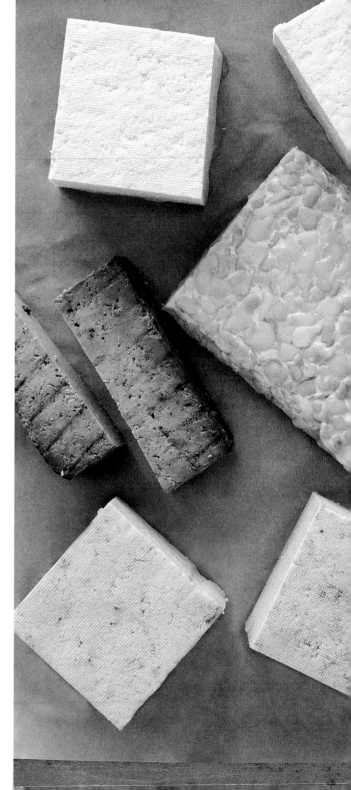

You see boring tofu bricks. I see tons of potential!

starter kit recipe: simple seared tofu

Cube 4 to 6 ounces firm tofu and pat it dry. Place a wok or sauté pan over medium-high heat and add 1 teaspoon of olive oil and a drop of roasted sesame oil. When hot, add the tofu, ½ teaspoon chopped garlic, and ½ teaspoon minced fresh or jarred ginger. Sear for several minutes, until golden on one side, then flip and sear on the other side. Add a big side of stir-fried snow peas and mushrooms and an optional ½ cup cooked soba (buckwheat) noodles. Sprinkle with chopped green onions and a little reduced-sodium soy sauce or Bragg Liquid Aminos. You're set!

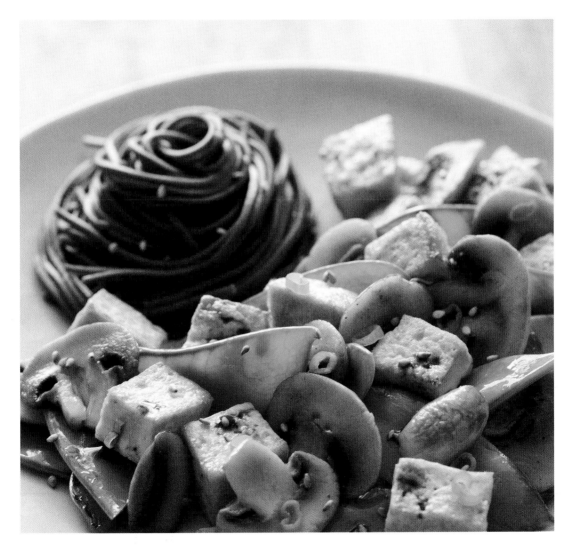

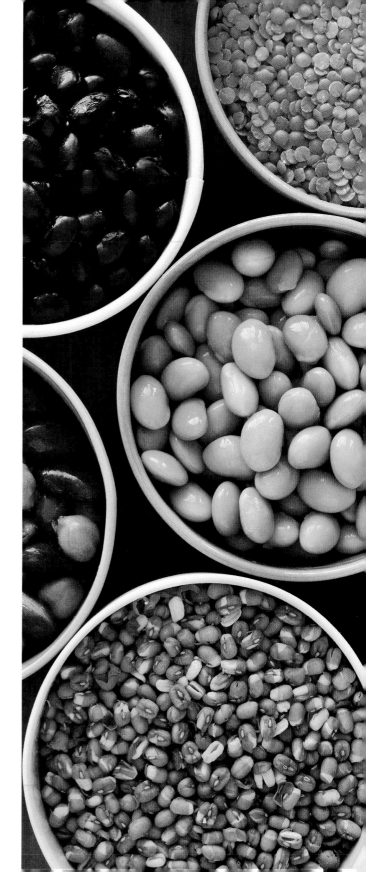

Your Life on the B-List: Beans!

Eat them: 2 to 3 times a week
A serving is: ¾ to 1 cup cooked

Beans get a big exclamation point because, to me, they're the unsung heroes of our diets. If diets were a movie, beans would be B-list actors with A-list impact—they deserve way more credit for the good they do. After all, beans and legumes are cheap, versatile, delicious, and loaded with protective nutrients, plant-based proteins, minerals, and fiber.

You also have so much variety to choose from: lentils (brown or black), mung beans (you gotta try 'em!), edamame, black beans, cannellini beans, chickpeas—any beans are on my A-list.

Of course, what everyone thinks about first when they hear the word "beans" are the complex oligosaccharides that travel largely unchanged through the upper intestine but are readily consumed by microorganisms in the digestive tract (specifically, *Methanobrevibacter smithii*), which produce volumes of methane called flatus . . .

Okay, I hear you: "Can it, nutrition girl—beans give me gas!"

Ah, but I'm gonna show you how to bypass that . . . keep reading.

MY EASY STRATEGY FOR BEANS:

1. Get 'em to go. Buy a quart of beans to go from your local Mexican fast-food joint. Most offer pinto, black, or both, in vegetarian forms (meaning no lard), and the best part is that the restaurant has done all the work, from degassing to cooking. For just a few dollars a quart, you'll have 4 to 5 servings. Now all you need are some sautéed fajita-style veg and you've got dinner—and leftovers (see the recipe on page 130).

2. Try this quick fix: Lentils and mung beans are my ultimate fave because they're easier to cook than rice (see the recipe below).

3. Or this even *quicker* fix: Score sprouted lentils or mung beans from a health food store. These are literally ready in five minutes, and since they're sprouted, they're easier to digest. Plus, they're super cheap.

4. Pop open a can. Make sure to get the ones labeled "BPA free" when you have the option (the lining of most cans contains this potentially harmful chemical), and drain and rinse them to knock down the sodium content *and* degas them. Toss them in soups, on salads, or into a breakfast burrito. Tip: Keep them in your pantry so you always have a protein backup.

starter kit recipe:
lentils or mung beans

Super easy! And beans are so delicious and nutritious, I'm sure you'll put them on your A-list in no time. You can cook mung beans the same way.

MAKES APPROXIMATELY 3 SERVINGS

1 cup petite or regular lentils
2½ cups low-sodium broth

Combine the lentils and broth in a medium pot and bring to a boil. Reduce the heat, cover, and simmer until tender, 20 to 25 minutes. Drain.

Get Cracking: Omega-3–Rich Eggs

Eat them: 2 to 3 times a week
A serving is: 4 to 6 whites or 1 whole egg plus 3 to 5 whites

Many people still believe these oval guys are evil—Not true! Eggs are the *good* guys—they just need a better publicist. (Sorry, that's how we talk in LA.)

For starters, research has linked egg consumption to weight loss. The yolks are also loaded with choline, a nutrient that fights inflammation and boosts brain function. (So is that why smart people are called "eggheads"? Hmm.)

What about the cholesterol? I've got good news for you: Research shows that it's the saturated fat more than the actual cholesterol in our food that bumps up your levels. So I recommend going moderate on the yolks, with three to four a week (but knock yourself out with the egg whites).

Most important, make sure the carton says the eggs are "omega-3 enhanced" or "enriched" (it has to do with how the hens are fed). They cost a little more than regular eggs, but they're still a great deal for protein.

Since the yolk is what contains the omega-3s, you can save money by mixing one whole omega-3 egg with three-plus regular egg whites.

And *hello*—is there a more versatile food on the planet? Eggs can show up for breakfast, lunch, or dinner.

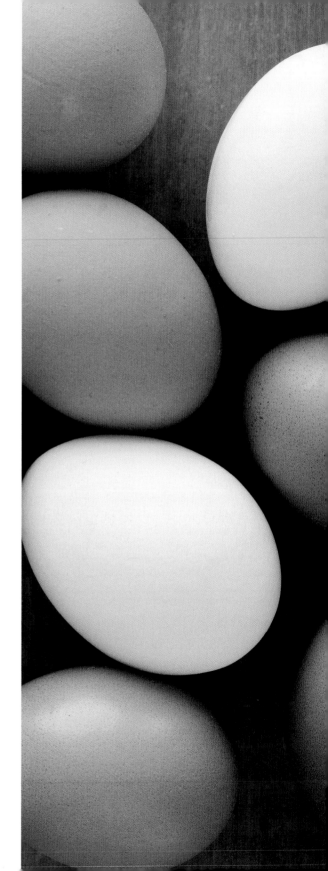

starter kit recipe: egg white-*ish* salad

When you think eggs, think beyond breakfast! My famous Egg White-*ish* Salad was a kitchen staple at the *Biggest Loser* ranch. It makes for a perfect quick meal that doesn't involve a drive-thru.

MAKES ¼ TO ½ CUP FOR SNACK, ¾ TO 1 CUP FOR LUNCH

- **12 hard-boiled egg whites**
- **3 hard-boiled egg yolks**
- **2 tablespoons reduced-fat Vegenaise or reduced-fat mayo**
- **¼ cup chopped red onion or fresh chives**
- **⅛ teaspoon turmeric (optional)**
- **½ teaspoon mustard**
- **⅛ teaspoon paprika (optional)**

Chop or grate the egg whites and yolks and place them in a bowl. Stir in the Vegenaise, onion, turmeric, if using, and mustard. Top with the paprika, if using. Prep a batch so it's always within reach for weekday lunches or snacks.

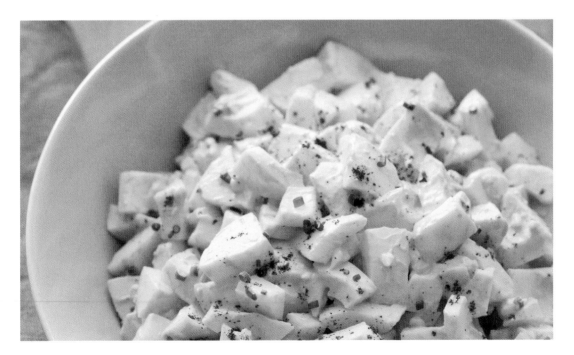

The Little Three—Chicken, Turkey, and Beef (Formerly the Big Three)

Eat them: 2 to 4 times a week
A serving is: 3 to 5 ounces (cooked)

You don't need me to tell you what to do with chicken, turkey, and grass-fed beef, right? Or any other type of meat, for that matter. You probably own dozens of cookbooks that feature dozens of recipes. Just remember that 1 serving should be just 3 to 5 ounces. (And do you need a dietitian to tell you that deep-fried chicken and gravy-smothered turkey are not your friends?)

Follow my Protein GPS system, and over time I'll bet that you won't even notice you're eating so much less poultry and beef. In fact, most people stop craving it altogether!

So there you have it: fourteen meals. Down. Done!

Sound Bite: Hey, What About Cheese?

Yes, cheese *is* a source of protein. But here's my take on the stuff: Cheese offers a huge flavor punch, which means you can use a small amount *as a snack or a condiment only*, rather than a main ingredient. (Adios, quesadillas.) Stick to servings that are no more than an ounce.

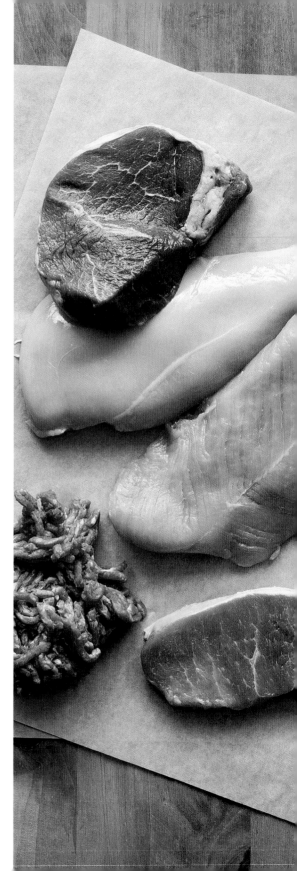

STEP 3: Have a little healthy fat—yes, I *insist*.

Please don't go all fat-free on me! While all the veggies you're eating are good for you, they're even better with a *mandatory* touch of good fat, such as olive oil or avocado to maximize your nutrient absorption. Healthy oils make you feel full longer too. Just pick one per meal. Some options and serving amounts:

- 1 to 2 teaspoons of oil (40 to 80 calories). My classic go-tos are cold-pressed extra virgin olive oil, avocado and walnut oils (for salads and marinades) and extra light or pure olive oil, for high-heat cooking.

- A yummy bottled salad dressing (no more than 80 calories in 2 tablespoons—see page 190 for suggestions). And don't buy fat-free! Those dressings are less real than *The Real Housewives of Orange County*.

- ¼ avocado (60 calories)

- 1 tablespoon prepared pesto sauce (approximately 60 calories)

- 1 or 2 teaspoons chia or flaxseed oil (40 calories per teaspoon)

Sound Bite: The Devil Is in the Dressing.

Picture this: liquefied fried chicken. Would you pour that on your salad? No way! But get this:

Your typical restaurant salad comes drenched in a minimum of *4 tablespoons* of dressing. Even the average salad bar ladle doles out that much. So either way, you're getting around 340 calories and your RDA (recommended *decade* allowance) of fat with the dressing alone. That's like chowing down an order of extra crispy. Some dressings have saturated fat, so you're essentially pouring concrete straight into your arteries and molding it onto your hips and thighs. In Hollywood, people are now bringing their dressings to work and even to restaurants. Sounds over the top, but it's a genius trend to follow! Or ask for dressing on the side with some lemon wedges—then squeeze the juice in to dilute it. To get the most out of a small amount of dressing, the key is to toss, toss, toss! If you toss thoroughly, the dressing gets distributed really well and no leaf goes undressed.

- 1 tablespoon chia seeds or ground flaxseed (40 to 65 calories)

- 1 tablespoon chopped walnuts or slivered almonds (about 50 calories)—this is not an add-on, it's *in lieu* of salad dressing!

- 1 tablespoon reduced-fat mayo (45 calories)

- 2 tablespoons guacamole or hummus mixed with 2 tablespoons lime or lemon juice (50 to 70 calories)—it's the ultimate all-natural dip or dressing

STEP 4: Don't go against the grain! Use my Slice Trick to cut your carbs.

I confess: I have cravings too—and they're not for eggplant or tofu. (Even *I* think that's weird.) Like many people, mine are usually for something soft-baked, chewy, or crunchy.

Yes, I have an inner cookie monster.

So I totally understand your craving for carb yumminess. And let me be the first to tell you that it's perfectly okay! I'm not one of those carb-o-phobic dietitians who go all Atkins on you. There are plenty of healthy options—and they *belong* in your diet.

The problem? Carbs are the food group people most overeat. In my practice, I hear a lot of "Quinoa is healthy! Brown rice is good for you!" And that's true, of course. But healthy doesn't mean *all you can eat.* As I mentioned in the beginning of this chapter, even though the *Biggest Loser* contestants had switched to better foods by the time I showed up, they were still piling between 400 and 600 calories on their plates *just* in carbs!

Here's my secret to success when dishing out carbs: **Think in bread slices!** All my patients and show contestants still use this trick all the time—works wonders for portion control. From now on, when you select a carb (even the healthiest of the healthiest), I want you to mentally compare your portion to a typical piece of sandwich bread—and envision how many slices you've got on your plate. My Slice Trick works like this:

This Serving of Carbs = X Slices of Bread

Or, to give you a specific example:

This ⅓-cup serving of brown rice = 1 slice of whole wheat bread

Now, the average amount of brown rice I see on most plates is 1 cup. That's three slices of bread at one sitting. If you want to lose weight, you might rethink that!

Here are some handy carb equivalents using my Slice Trick—they're your guide to knowing what a healthy portion is:

1 SLICE OF BREAD (70 TO 90 CALORIES) =

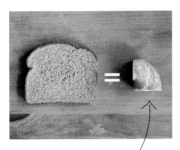

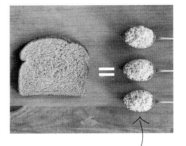

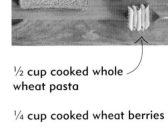

¼ whole wheat bagel (that's right, just a quarter of it!)

⅓ cup cooked brown rice

½ whole wheat pita

⅓ cup cooked quinoa

⅓ cup cooked farro

½ cup cooked whole wheat couscous

½ cup cooked whole wheat pasta

¼ cup cooked wheat berries

½ cup sweet potato (about half a smallish spud)

THE EX FACTOR: EXERCISE—AND HOW IT FITS INTO THE PLAN

You don't need me—the R.D.—to tell you that working out regularly (strength and cardio!) is important for weight loss. The question I always get is: Shouldn't I eat more if I'm active? My advice is that if you break a serious sweat most days of the week and find your stomach grumbling on the guidelines I've given you, you might need a morning or evening snack. You can also add a serving of carbs to your meal or go for the higher end of the suggested protein range. But watch how things go, scale-wise. Too often people use exercise as an excuse to eat more—and usually whatever they burned at the gym doesn't quite compensate for what they choose to "refuel" themselves with. So always ask yourself: Am I truly hungry? Or do I simply feel like I *deserve* to eat?

Sound Bite: Can't Wait to Lose Weight?

Want to fast-track your weight loss? Eat fiber-rich carbs at breakfast and maybe as a snack later—but skip them at lunch and/or dinner. Double up on veg and you will barely notice they're missing. But your scale will!

YOUR FLIP-IT METHOD CHEAT SHEET

- Build every lunch and dinner with a minimum of 1½ to 2 cups of veg.

- Add a lean protein according to my weekly 14-meal Protein GPS:
    - 4 meals with low-mercury, high–omega-3 fish
    - 2 or 3 meals with beans
    - 2 meals with tofu
    - 2 or 3 meals with eggs

  That leaves 2 to 4 meals for chicken, turkey, grass-fed beef, or other lean protein.

- Limit good fats to 40 to 80 calories per meal. They're important to have, but I've gotta give you some parameters!

- Have an *optional* serving of a whole grain carb. Use my Slice Trick to keep portions in check.

- Always do your best to apply the Flip-It Method—but if you find yourself eating in unfamiliar territory, just remember that lunch and dinner should be roughly 400 to 550 calories. Don't get all type-A about it—just keep in mind my favorite rule: It's not what you do *sometimes*, but what you do *most of the time* that makes a difference.

- Now **go shopping! Jump to Part 3 to get started!**

snacks are for losers— *weight* losers!

Between-meal bites screw up sooo many diets, unless you do them *right*

Dieters all think they know the Enemy:

It's the cheesecake. *Evil temptress!*

The white rice that came with their takeout. *Empty-carb alert.*

The apple juice. *Liquid candy!*

And please—don't even get them started on snacks.

"Come on, Rachel," they say. "I'm trying to lose weight here—I can't afford to snack! Aren't those extra calories the first thing I should ditch?"

No way. If you're trying to lose weight, you actually can't afford *not* to snack. When you skip it, you'll nibble thoughtlessly throughout the day—or you'll get too hungry and go overboard at mealtime. (Think grizzly bear at a Vegas buffet.) Either way, your odds of losing weight will fall somewhere between nada and zero.

Here's an example of how easy it is for even a super-smart, super-educated person to fall into the "it's too small to count" trap—and wind up grazing on way more than she would have if she'd had planned-out, "Rachel-approved" snacks.

The Ph.D. (Partially Healthy Diet) Doesn't Make the Grade

I have this patient who's a brilliant professor, but she can't lose weight. So as I do in all my initial consultations, I have her fill me in on what's filling her up.

This professor tells me, "Rachel, I eat salads, I play tennis, I'm on my feet most of the day. And I no longer hit the office vending machine—I just stick to my meals and that's it. I haven't the slightest clue why the pounds aren't coming off!" She's trying to show me what a good girl she's been. And that's typical. No one comes into my office and says, "I'm a chain donut eater. Why can't I lose weight?"

But as I hear about all this angelic behavior, I'm thinking, *Okay, what's the whole story? Where's everything in between?* I know that 90 percent of the time the problem is something my patients do that they don't think about. So I start poking around for clues—call it *Beverly Hills CSI: Caloric Sources Investigation.*

Little by little (make that bite by bite) the truth comes spilling out. First, I learn that the good professor likes to shop at a warehouse store that offers great deals on my recommended foods. Nothing wrong with that. But the store also offers food samples—and they're tiny nibbles, so they're harmless, right?

Then she gets home and unloads the groceries. She sees an empty pizza box that her husband left behind. Well, not really empty. He left two crusts, and it would be a shame to just throw those out—and they're leftovers, so they're harmless, right?

Then she starts making dinner. She's having salad, but the kids want mac and cheese, and she has to taste it to know when it's ready—just small tastes, really, so they're harmless, right?

And while she's in the kitchen, she also makes the kids' lunches for the next day (PB&J). But, like their father, they also don't like crusts, so she eats those too . . .

It doesn't take a Ph.D. to see what's going wrong here, right?

The professor didn't factor in all those extra calories because, in her mind, they were completely insignificant—not even worth the ink to write in her diet log. But guess what? Those nibbles seriously added up (see the box on page 61)! If I had had a hidden camera following her around, she'd be horrified by her own reality show: Every day she's consuming *an entire fourth meal* consisting of small but calorie-dense bites.

You don't have to officially sit down to a giant, buttercream-frosted cupcake to commit diet homicide. A taste here, a bite there, and any hope of weight loss is dead.

What do you do?

I'll show you how to get this snack thing right, so your between-meal bites actually become your fast track to weight loss.

EXTRA BITES BECOME MEGA-BITES!

Get a load of the diet homicide you commit just by tasting and nibbling throughout the day.

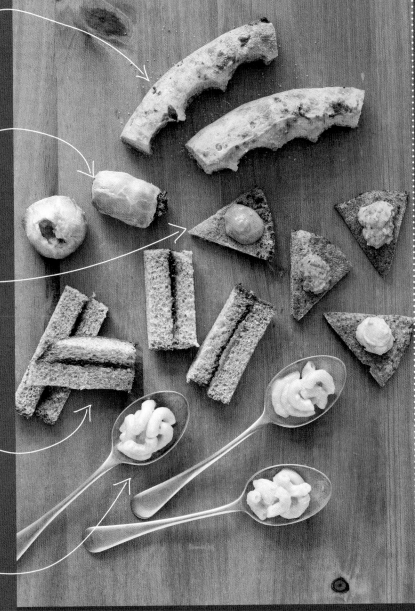

YOU THINK: *This isn't eating, really—I'm just cleaning up here.*

YOU JUST ATE: 128 calories! Did you say . . . "cleaning" or "hauling"?

YOU THINK: *Two mini bite-size nothings.*

YOU JUST ATE: Roughly 140 calories. Bite-size nothings can add up to boat-size somethings.

YOU THINK: *I have to sample all four flavors of hummus. After all, it's healthy!*

YOU JUST ATE: 132 calories of "healthy." That's not what I call sampling!

YOU THINK: *It's just the crust with a little PB&J. It's basically trash. And trash doesn't have calories.*

YOU JUST ATE: 130 calories—and last I checked, 130 is greater than zero.

YOU THINK: *I should see if the pasta's ready. Oh, and I need to check the seasoning. I'll just steal another spoonful.*

YOU JUST ATE: Those spoonfuls add up to 80 calories. So theft isn't the only crime you're committing. You just killed your diet!

TOTAL CALORIES FROM THOSE EXTRA BITES: 610!
That's a fourth—but super-unsatisfying—meal.

How to snack—the *smart* way!

You have three snack time slots throughout the day:

1. Your optional a.m. snack
2. Your *mandatory* p.m. snack (between lunch and dinner)
3. A strictly optional after-dinner treat

Snacks are the one big exception to my no-calorie-counting rule. You *must* keep close tabs on them, or you can go wrong—as in, extra-pants-size wrong.

So stick within the calorie ranges I'll be giving you. But here's the bright (and tasty) side: You will still have a wealth of options! Not only will you get through the day without a grumbly stomach (and attitude to match), you'll also tune your body to weight-loss mode.

A.M. (Alternative Munching) Snack:
Enjoy an *optional* midmorning bite that's under 100 calories.

I call this snack optional because after a balanced, high-fiber breakfast, you'll likely make it all the way to lunch without getting hungry. Plus, that gap between breakfast and lunch is shorter than the one between lunch and dinner, so if you can skip it, skip it!

In fact, research shows that most people eat midmorning snacks not because they're hungry but because they're bored ("I hate Mondays!") or the food is just sitting there tempting them ("Hello, beautiful, my name is chocolate-glazed donut!").

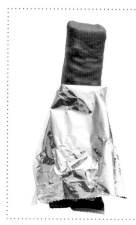

TIME TO *LOWER* THE BAR!

When did we all become so obsessed with snack bars? Most of the time they're just a bunch of grains heavily processed with some kind of sugar and a lab full of mystery ingredients. Yet they've got their own supermarket aisle now! The need for portability, I understand. But you can throw together something just as handy—and a bazillion times healthier. (See Grab-n-Go Snacks on page 76.)

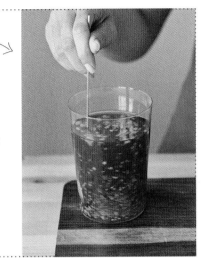

Try this!

MY TRICK OF THE TRADE

Curb midmorning or afternoon cravings (vending machine raid!) and earn yourself serious skinny bonus points by sipping some chia seeds stirred into a glass of iced tea or water with a splash of pomegranate juice. The seeds won't dissolve, but you won't really taste them. Just be sure to count the calories (even though they're small) toward your snack.

If you genuinely *do* need a snack (maybe you worked out or ate breakfast super-early), think within the 100-calories-or-fewer range. Some ideas:

- Celery sticks with 1 wedge of Laughing Cow light cheese
- 1 hard-boiled egg
- 1 piece of fruit, such as a small apple, orange, banana, or 1 cup of berries
- ½ cup nonfat Greek yogurt
- 1 stick low-fat string cheese
- 10 almonds
- Baby carrots with 2 tablespoons salsa
- Sliced cucumbers with 1 tablespoon hummus

P.M. (Positively Mandatory) Snack:
Tame your inner "bread-ator" with a 150- to 175-calorie midday snack.

Want to lose weight and not feel hungry? Then this snack is thoroughly *nonnegotiable.* You have too many hours between lunch and dinner, and if you don't eat a little something by the time dinner rolls around, you'll feel like the world owes you food—and lots of it.

And that's when you see the Enemy: that basket staring back at you from the middle of the table. Sometimes at lunch, sometimes dinner, but always there.

This basket comes filled with bread—or the even more wicked fried tortilla chips. They'll tempt you even when you're not hungry, so when you're famished, your powers of resistance become as stable as a soap bubble. You can almost hear it pop! "Just a bite" or "just one" quickly turns into a fatty carbo-fest. Look:

MINI FOOD AUTOPSY ALERT: BREAD!

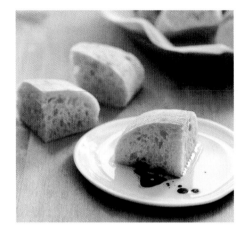

Feast your eyes (not your mouth) on this: bread squares—smaller than what you'll find in a typical restaurant—soaked like a sponge in a wading pool of olive oil and vinegar. Those three small pieces add up to . . . drum roll, please . . . 345 calories! No joke. That's not a snack: That's a calorie bomb.

To tame your inner bread-ator and avoid *Attack the basket or death!* mode, eat your afternoon snack. Don't go all martyr on me and think you'll "save" calories and lose weight faster if you pass it up. Trust me: Skipping the p.m. snack always backfires.

SUPER-CRITICAL NOTE: The type of snack you choose really matters! Here are the rules:

1. Your snack needs to satisfy and fill you up. When was the last time you ate one of those 100-calorie cracker packs and thought, *Okay, I'm full!* Total LOL. More like, "*This* tiny thing is supposed to hold me until dinner?!"

2. It needs to be *balanced*. Ideally a combination of protein, fiber, and some good fat to keep your blood sugar steady and control hunger for hours.

3. Take care of your carbo-urges here. If you're taking the speedy weight-loss route and not having carbs at lunch or dinner, use this p.m. snack to feed your craving. Since the range of calories is limited, you can't go overboard. This is my ultimate trick of the trade for staying on track and not feeling deprived.

4. Also think: fruit! Snacks are the perfect time for it (aside from breakfast, of course). And I don't know why, but no one ever thinks to grab an apple anymore—it's always trail mix or a bar. But fruit is just as portable and gives you a hit of fiber that's way more satisfying than a dinky processed bar. My faves: apples, tangerines, pears, oranges, and berries. But they're all good!

5. Be creative. Sure, some baby carrots and a string cheese make a perfectly fine snack. But you can do better than that Diet 101 basic. Think of yourself as a fashion consultant with a tight budget. You can have fun assembling outfits as long as you don't exceed the caloric limits.

These Mini Meals Are Caloric Steals

Here are a few "outfits" to stimulate your imagination—and prove that you can do a lot within that 150- to 175-calorie range!

Add as much veg as you like to any of the snacks.
Those calories don't count—so go all out!

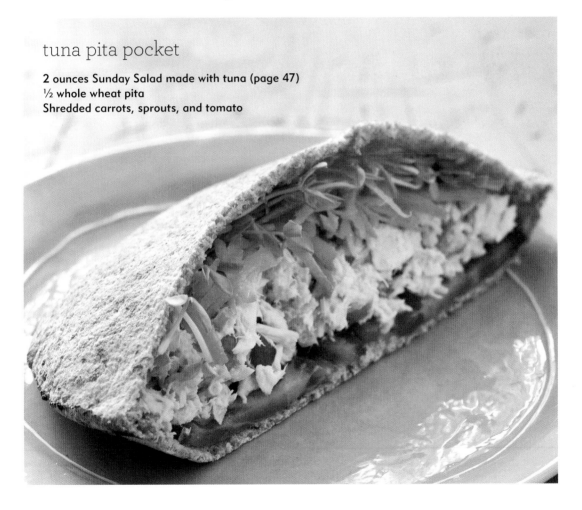

tuna pita pocket

2 ounces Sunday Salad made with tuna (page 47)
½ whole wheat pita
Shredded carrots, sprouts, and tomato

toaster-oven tortilla pizza

1 sprouted or whole wheat tortilla (approximately 80 cal)
¼ cup marinara sauce
1 ounce reduced-fat Mexican cheese blend
Sliced mushrooms, red onion, and grape tomatoes (or any other veg)

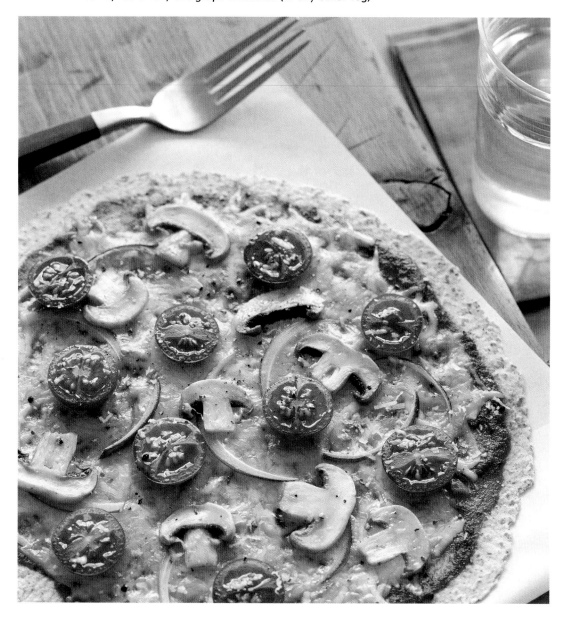

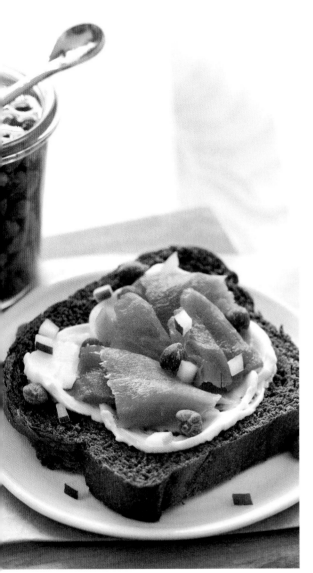

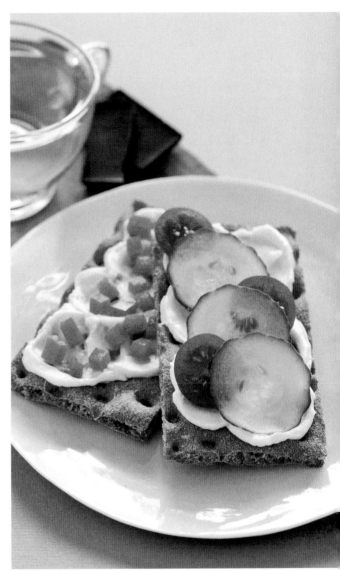

better than a bagel and lox

1 slice pumpernickel bread
1 wedge Laughing Cow Light cheese
1 ounce smoked salmon
Diced red onion
A sprinkling of capers

the 3-cs: crackers, cheese, and chocolate

2 Wasa crackers
1 wedge Laughing Cow Light cheese
Top with any veg you like!
1 premeasured 50-calorie chocolate square

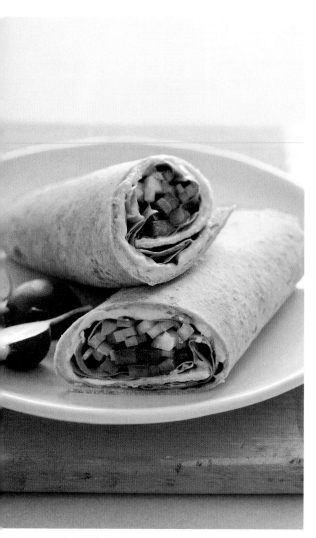

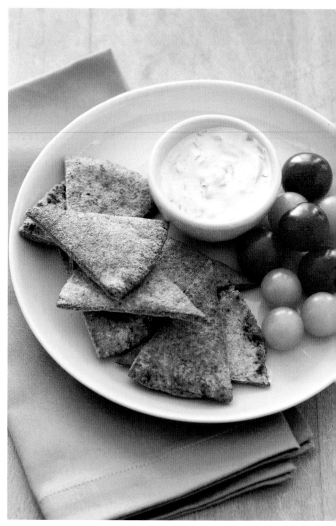

loaded hummus wrap

1 sprouted or whole wheat tortilla
   (approximately 80 cal)
2 tablespoons hummus
Shredded carrots, baby spinach,
   cucumbers, and bell pepper strips

tzatziki with veggies and toasted pita wedges

2 tablespoons low-fat prepared tzatziki dip
1 whole wheat pita, cut into wedges and toasted
Cherry tomatoes

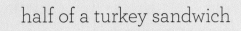

half of a turkey sandwich

1 slice Ezekiel bread
2 ounces nitrate-free turkey
1 teaspoon mustard
Lettuce and tomato

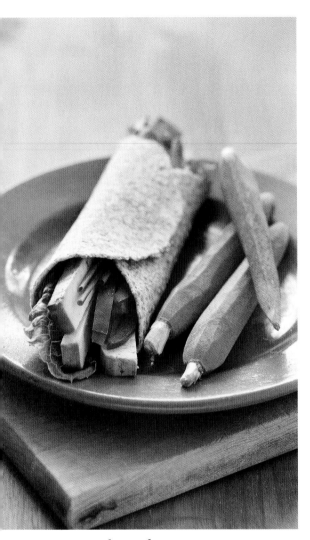

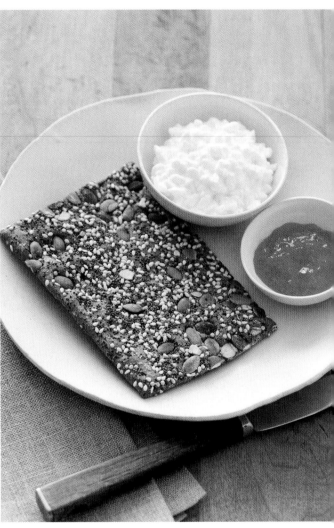

teriyaki tofu wrap with crudités

2 ounces teriyaki-flavored tofu
One 6- to 8-inch whole wheat tortilla
Lettuce and bell pepper strips
Side of baby carrots

jammin' flatbread

1 Doctor Kracker crispbread
¼ cup low-fat cottage cheese
1 tablespoon naturally sweetened jam

cheesy black bean soup

1 cup vegetable black bean soup
1 tablespoon reduced-fat Mexican cheese blend, melted into the soup

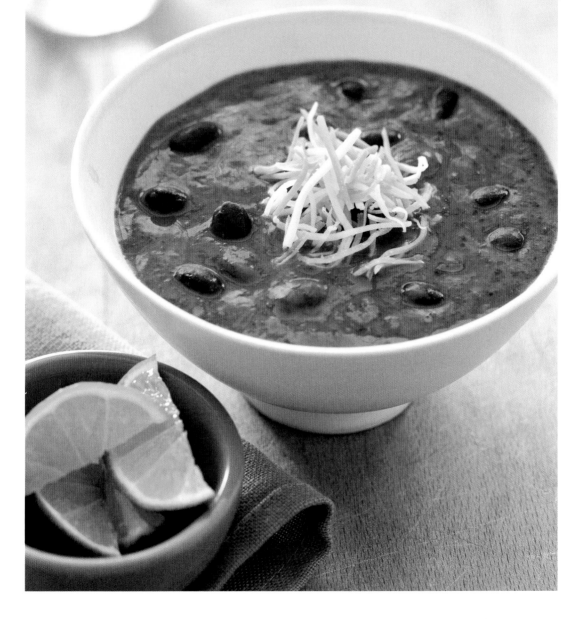

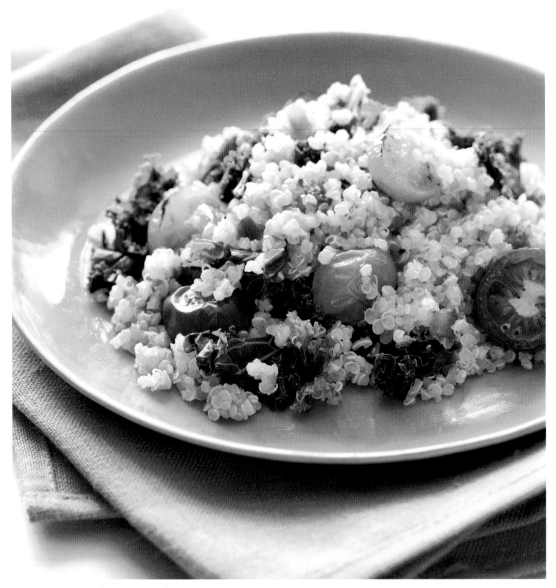

quinoa with mixed veggies

²/₃ **cup cooked quinoa**
Cooked tomatoes, red onion, and kale or broccoli florets
Juice from ¹/₄ **lemon**

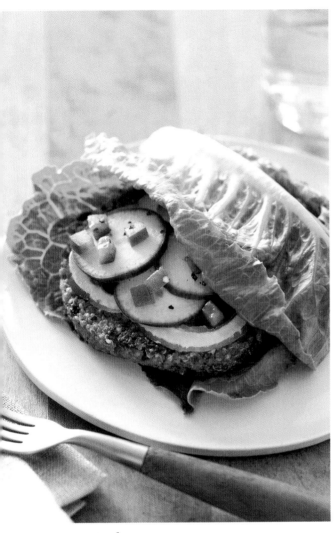

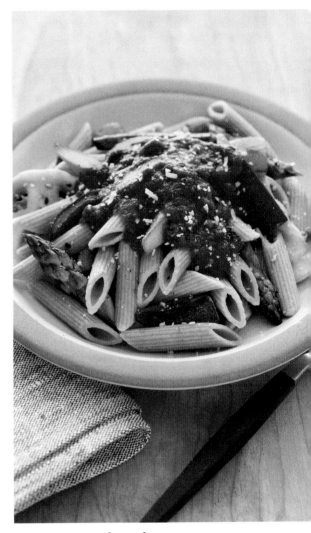

veggie burger wrap

1 cooked veggie burger patty
3 lettuce leaves
Sliced tomato, red onion, and cucumber
Reduced-fat dressing or mustard (optional)

mini pasta bowl

¾ cup whole wheat pasta
¼ cup marinara sauce
1 teaspoon grated Parmesan cheese
Any veg you like!

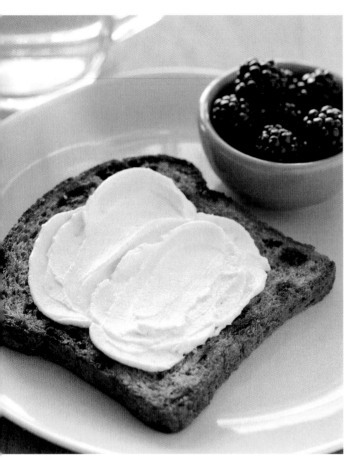

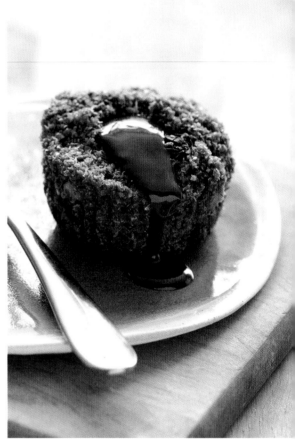

toasted raisin bread
with goat cheese

1 slice Ezekiel sprouted raisin bread
2 tablespoons soft goat cheese
½ cup blackberries

chocolate lava fiber cake

1 mini fiber cake (Zen Bakery or Trader
  Joe's, or my recipe, page 98)
One premeasured 50-calorie dark chocolate
  square, melted on top

skinny mineral-rich wrap

2 ounces Sunday Salad made with salmon (page 47)
2 nori seaweed sheets (packed with minerals!)
Any veg you like

GRAB-N-GO SNACKS

Always on the run? Don't fall for those softball-size muffins at the coffee shop. (Plus, who has time for those lines?) Pack a few of these snacks in advance so you can just snag one on your way out the door.

1 Wasa cracker
Mixed vegetables
3 tablespoons hummus

120 calories

2 cups strawberries
1 square dark chocolate

145 calories

10 crackers
1 cheese

155 calories

1 cup Kamut Puffs
½ cup freeze-dried berries
1 hard-boiled egg

160 calories

30 pistachios
1 cheese

150 calories

Low-carb tortilla
2 ounces turkey
Vegetables
Mustard

130 calories

2 Wasa crackers
1 cheese spread

105 calories

14 almonds
1 cheese

160 calories

Snack-tastrophes!

You know your greatest weakness: That snack item (maybe items) that make you throw all limits out the window. I'm not talking cookies, chips, or other addictive junk. I'm talking foods that are good in small doses but that so many people overeat. I call them "bloopers."

Classic blooper #1: Peanut butter overload!

Yes, it's healthy at 1 tablespoon per serving, but I rarely come across a patient who precisely measures 1 tablespoon of PB, levels it off with a knife, does not lick, and returns the excess to the jar. Most "tablespoons" look like the iceberg that sank the Titanic. The spoon is practically bending in half! And once you spread that mound of peanutty goodness on toast or an apple, you're plunging mouth-first into 300-plus calories. Classic!

See that tiny container on the left that's half full? That's 1 tablespoon of PB; the full container has 2 tablespoons of it—yep, that's 180 calories in just a mouthful! When I showed this to *The Biggest Loser* contestants, they went nuts. So do this: Buy 1-tablespoon (not 2) premeasured pouches of nut butter. Or be totally type-A meticulous and, when you get the jar home, preportion 1-tablespoon servings into mini salad-dressing cups, so they're ready to go and you bypass the straight-from-the-container pitfall. Keeping that peanut butter jar out of reach will keep your diet goals within reach.

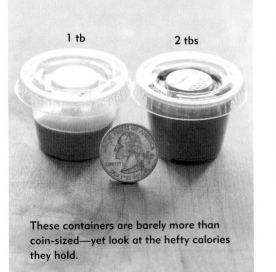

1 tb   2 tbs

These containers are barely more than coin-sized—yet look at the hefty calories they hold.

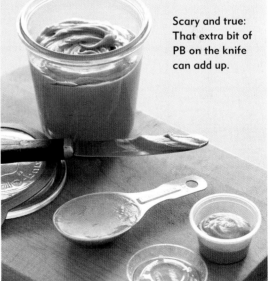

Scary and true: That extra bit of PB on the knife can add up.

Classic blooper #2: Thinking "healthy" means "eat all you want."

You may be thinking, *duh*—peanut butter is a blooper waiting to happen! Anything that luscious must be approached with caution. You, on the other hand, are a healthy snacker: almonds, kale chips, nonfat smoothies.

That's great, but "good for you" doesn't mean "go to town." Just because something's labeled organic, vegan, heart-healthy, all-natural, nonfat, or gluten-free, don't be fooled into believing your bathroom scale won't notice. Bag of almonds? Very nutritious—but if you dip your hand into it three times a day, you're adding about 450 calories to your diet (the caloric equivalent of a cheeseburger)! And don't get me started on smoothies, which are entire meals sucked through a straw.

Check out the pics below: I grabbed these snacks at a health food store. In these portions, eating hand-to-mouth will only add inches to your waist!

Bottom line: Watch the calories in your snacks—even the angelic ones. And calorie counts can vary from brand to brand, so pay attention!

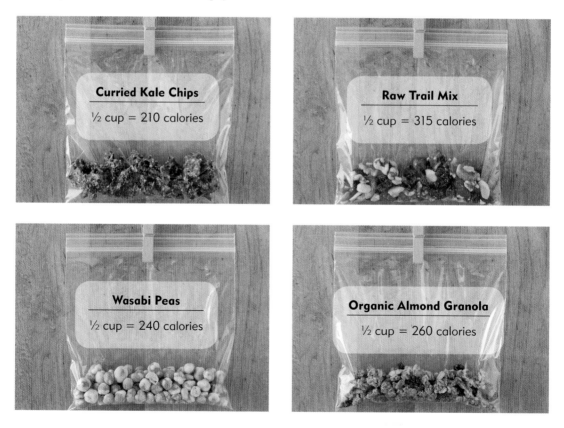

Curried Kale Chips
½ cup = 210 calories

Raw Trail Mix
½ cup = 315 calories

Wasabi Peas
½ cup = 240 calories

Organic Almond Granola
½ cup = 260 calories

YOU CAN BEND THE RULES A BIT AT SNACK TIME

Call it your Flexible Food Fix. An eating plan should never feel extreme in any way, because eventually you'll walk away from it. That's why fad diets never work! Since there's no denying that we all get cravings, I say: Feed the need occasionally at snack time.

Let's say you really want a not-so-perfect bread (no visible grains), a frozen treat (a little higher in sugar), or some other snack item. Better to satisfy your craving in mini form with your calorie-controlled snack than with an 800-calorie mega-wrap for lunch—or a full-blown ice cream sundae. Because of the narrow margin of calories, you can't mess up big.

Again, remember my mantra: It's what you do *most* of the time, not some of the time that makes a difference. Consider this snack your Flexible Food Fix of the day, and enjoy!

FRUIT AND NUTS 2.0

Since neither of these guys come with handy Nutrition Facts labels, how are you supposed to know if you're within the right calorie range? Use these guidelines for 100-calorie snack options and you'll always get it right.
(No bloopers for *you*!)

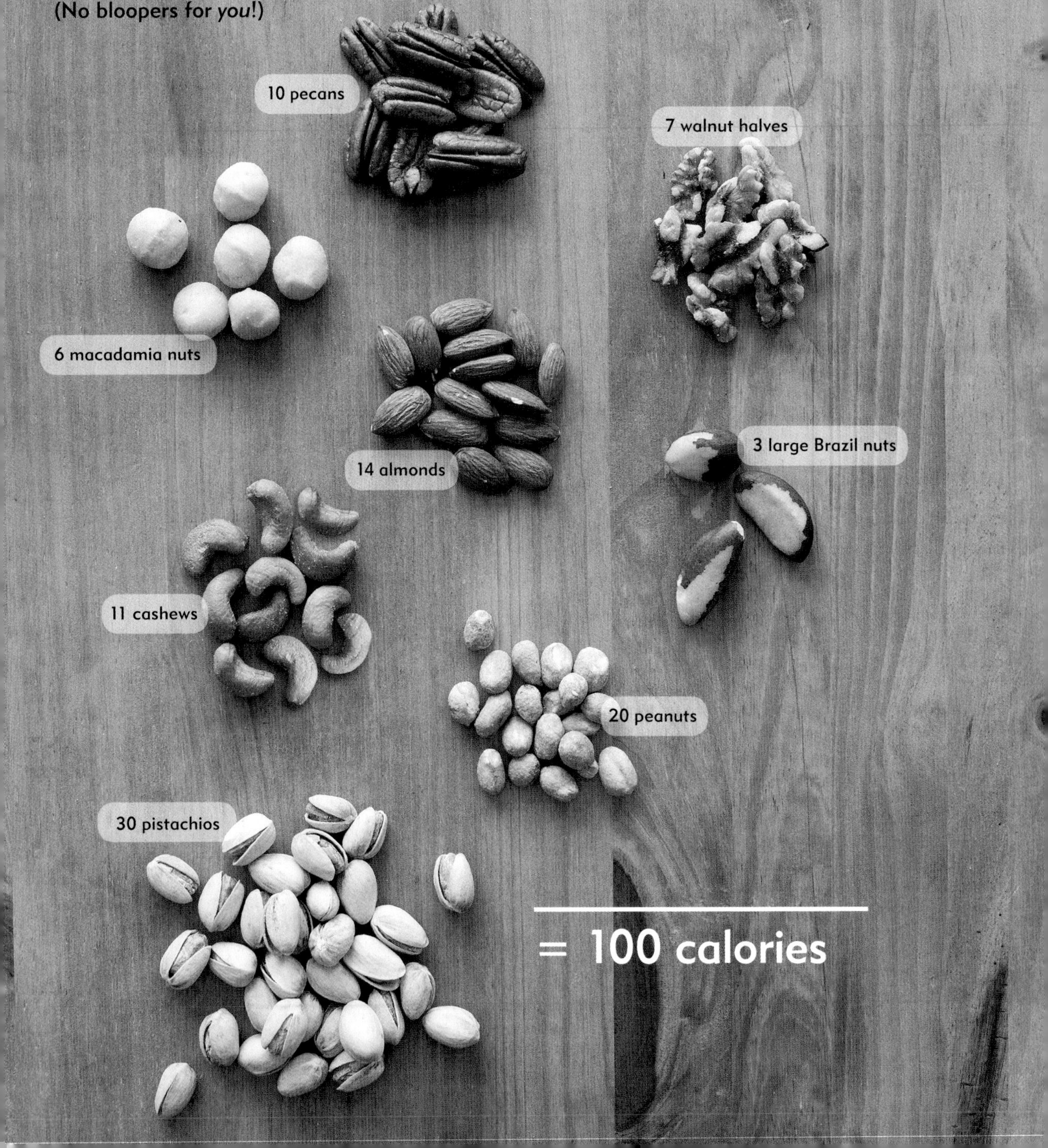

10 pecans

7 walnut halves

6 macadamia nuts

14 almonds

3 large Brazil nuts

11 cashews

20 peanuts

30 pistachios

= 100 calories

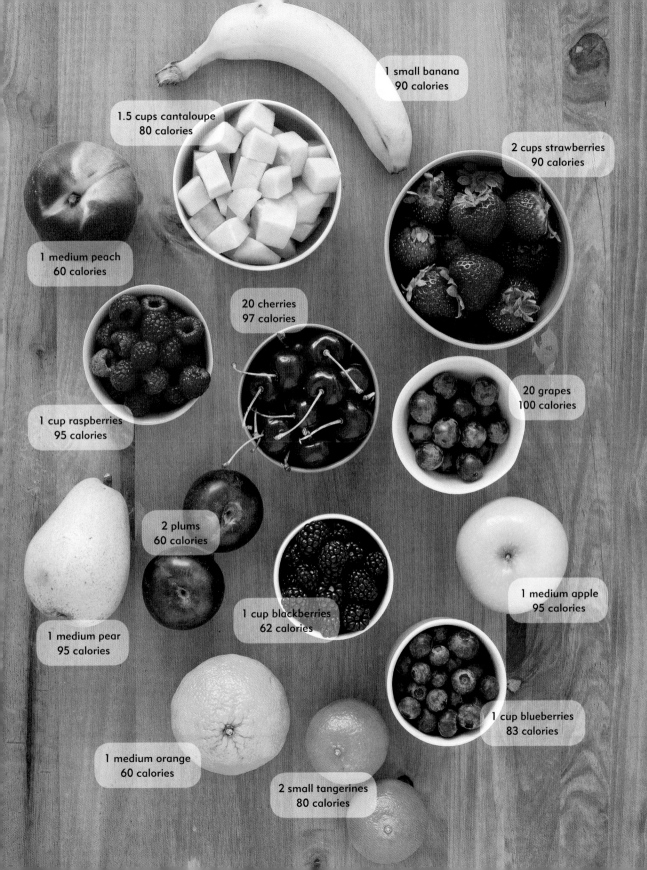

1 small banana
90 calories

1.5 cups cantaloupe
80 calories

2 cups strawberries
90 calories

1 medium peach
60 calories

20 cherries
97 calories

20 grapes
100 calories

1 cup raspberries
95 calories

2 plums
60 calories

1 medium apple
95 calories

1 cup blackberries
62 calories

1 medium pear
95 calories

1 cup blueberries
83 calories

1 medium orange
60 calories

2 small tangerines
80 calories

A.D. (After Dinner) Treat:
Savor an *optional* 100- to 150-calorie mini splurge

After dinner is total instinct time. The dishes and kids are put away . . . *ah,* chill time for yourself. So you're chatting with friends, watching a little TV, getting ready for the next day—and, instinctively, you want a snack to go with it.

Don't fight it, because instincts usually win. Just don't make it a habit.

Ideally, you should eat four times per day: breakfast, lunch, p.m. snack, dinner. So if you can do without this after-dinner treat, please try—especially if you want faster weight-loss results. I'm just giving you the *option.* From my experience, if I don't show people how to handle a craving, they'll go for it—and beyond. Before you can say, "Treat time!" they're drinking half a bottle of wine or eating straight out of the ice cream tub.

THE SECRET TO HEALTHY POPCORN? DIY

I *love* popcorn. It packs loads of fiber and more polyphenols (an antioxidant that may lower risk for heart disease and certain cancers) than many fruits and veg. But if you buy the microwavable bags at the store, often you'll get loads of junk to go with it: trans fats, artificial flavors, and a yellowish coating of artery-clogging fats. My solution? **DIY** for a snack that's just as fast and easy—and both organic and tasty. Added bonus: It's cheap! Even organic comes in at about **35 cents per serving**. All you have to do is:

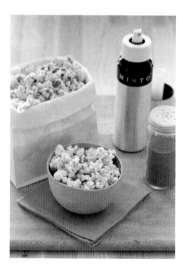

1. Put ¼ cup organic popcorn kernels in a brown paper lunch bag and fold the top over a few times.

2. Microwave, folded side up, for 2 to 3 minutes, until popping slows.

3. Mist the popcorn lightly with olive oil. (Use a Misto sprayer; see page 202.)

4. Add your own natural sweet or savory seasonings, such as:

   Ground Ceylon cinnamon (with an optional dash of palm sugar), nutritional yeast, grated Parmesan cheese, chili powder, dash of salt or garlic salt.

So here are some of my approved options for your after-dinner urges:

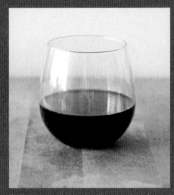

5.5-ounce glass of wine (with dinner, if you like—or after)

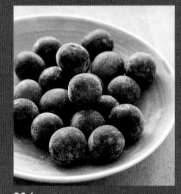

20 frozen grapes

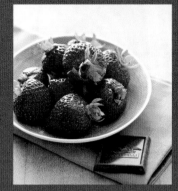

1 cup strawberries and 1 dark chocolate square

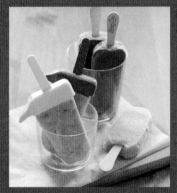

1 premeasured natural fudge or yogurt bar on a stick (absolutely no self-serve!)

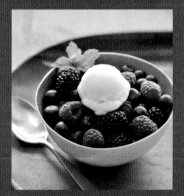

1 cup berries with ¼ cup mini-scoop of sorbet (great for dining in or out)

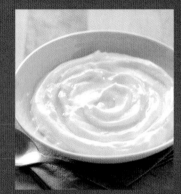

6 ounces nonfat Greek yogurt with 1 teaspoon naturally sweetened jam, honey, or maple syrup swirled in

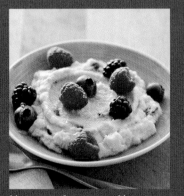

½ cup nonfat ricotta, ½ cup mixed berries, and a few drops of vanilla stevia or 1 teaspoon honey mixed together

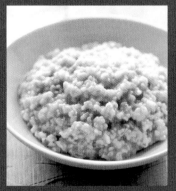

¾ cup cooked Scottish oatmeal with cinnamon (the melatonin in the oatmeal will help you sleep)

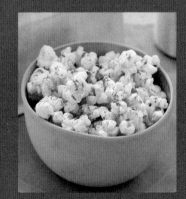

¼ cup popcorn kernels, popped the healthy way

NO JOKE: FROZEN DESSERTS THAT WON'T MAKE YOU SCREAM

Yes, we all scream for ice cream—but for anyone trying to lose weight, one look at the Nutrition Facts panel could be enough to make you scream. (And no, those nonfat options won't cut it.) But don't despair; I've got the ultimate ice cream alternatives.

Sinfully delicious 60-second fro-yo—it's easy!

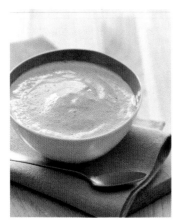

1. Put ¾ cup of nonfat Greek yogurt and 1 cup frozen berries in a bowl.

2. Add a few drops of a natural sweetener (I like vanilla-flavored stevia drops).

3. Whirl it up with an immersion blender and enjoy!

If you want a thicker texture, freeze it for 5 or 10 minutes. Oh, and it's only 120 to 150 calories, depending on which berries and yogurt you choose. No screaming necessary. Add one more step to make equally delicious frozen pops!

Creamy protein pops

1. Put 1 cup nonfat Greek yogurt and 1 cup thawed frozen berries (include the juice from the berries) in a bowl.

2. Add a few drops of stevia.

3. Mix with a spoon.

4. Scoop the mixture into 4 ice pop molds and freeze.

For approximately 50 calories and 6 grams of protein per frozen pop, it's a satisfying, low-sugar ice cream solution!

This dessert is ideal for those times when you're out with friends and they all want to hit the local fro-yo joint. Couldn't hurt, right? After all, it's the guilt-free dessert activity du jour. But get a load of this: Just one 8-ounce cup often contains a scary 52 grams of sugar and 240 calories—and that's *before* you hit the toppings bar! So much for "guilt-free."

How can you still join the party? Simple: Apply the Flip-It Method from the previous chapter! Rather than using the fro-yo as a base, start at the toppings bar and add your favorite fruit. Then swirl a little frozen yogurt on as the "topping." You'll satisfy that sweet tooth and bypass extra calories and a ton of sugar. Plus, you'll score added fiber and antioxidant power from the fruit.

The same Flip-It Method works in restaurants. A typical order of sorbet, for example, can cost you 300 calories—so flip it and ask for a bowl of berries with one small scoop of sorbet or a touch of whipped cream on top.

With the Flip-It Method, you'll never again be an outcast on a *deserted* island.

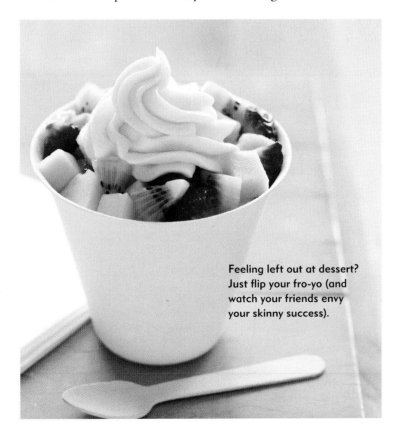

Feeling left out at dessert? Just flip your fro-yo (and watch your friends envy your skinny success).

YOUR SNACK CHEAT SHEET

- Have an *optional* a.m. snack that's 100 calories or less—and if you can skip it, skip it!

- Eat a *mandatory* p.m. snack that's 150 to 175 calories. Remember: This one's a must!

- Go for a mix of filling protein, fiber, and a touch of healthy fat.

- Watch calories! This is the one time I actually do want you to count them. It's key to keeping your snacks in check.

- Enjoy an after-dinner treat that's 100 to 150 calories. This is your chance to indulge a little. But know that you can fast-track weight loss if you can do without this snack.

- Make sure you always have healthy snack options on hand—**go shopping**! Check out the great options in Part 3.

let's eat

RECIPES FOR SUCCESS

10 days' worth of yummy mix-and-match meals

Like most Americans, I don't like being told what to do. Advice and suggestions? Absolutely—bring 'em on! Planning and coaching? We all need that. But dictated menus on exactly what I must eat three meals a day, seven days a week?

Forget about it.

I could never follow a rigid meal plan. What if I'm not in the mood for salmon Monday night? What if I'm traveling for work and can't make the high-fiber French toast for breakfast? It makes the plan harder to follow.

That's why I don't dictate them to my patients—and it's not just a matter of respecting adult independence. Regimented meal plans usually don't work. Even if you like routine and want everything planned out for you, you're more likely to fall off a nutritional plan unless you have some sense of choice and ownership. At some point you'll just say, "Aw, forget it!" (or some stronger expression) and pick up a four-cheese pizza and bread sticks on the way home.

So I created the following menus to let you pick and choose. I'm simply providing the first push on the swing to get you started! You'll still find specific ideas and simple recipes that follow my fiber rule for breakfast and the Flip-It Method and Protein GPS for lunch and dinner. But since the options at each meal (such as breakfast) contain roughly the same calories and follow the same principles, they're totally interchangeable.

I've also added some restaurant-friendly options, because I know you've got lunch meetings and nights when you can't be bothered to cook. You'll see how to navigate restaurant menus and make smart choices no matter where you pick up your fork.

A few guidelines: You'll notice a range of protein portions. Most women should stick to the low end; guys (or very tall or super-active women) should lean toward the high end. Lunches and dinners also have "optional" carb servings. If you want to expedite your weight loss, skip the carbs at one or both meals. Of course, I've given you some leeway to play around and see what works best for you. Each meal here makes one serving (unless otherwise noted), and you'll find many of the specific products I recommend starting in Part 3.

Bon appétit!

breakfast

By now you know that breakfast is by far the most important meal of the day. It's also the meal that presents so many options that are oh-so-wrong. Cheesecake pancakes, pork sausage, and a Coke? (A *real* option at one restaurant.) That's not a breakfast, that's a biohazard!

I've compiled for you several easy, *super-delicious* breakfasts, all designed to meet your a.m. fiber insurance. Think of it as a visual cheat sheet!

veggie-full omelet with goat cheese

Here's a tasty way to get your a.m. protein *and* fiber fix (it also works any time of day).

SERVES 1

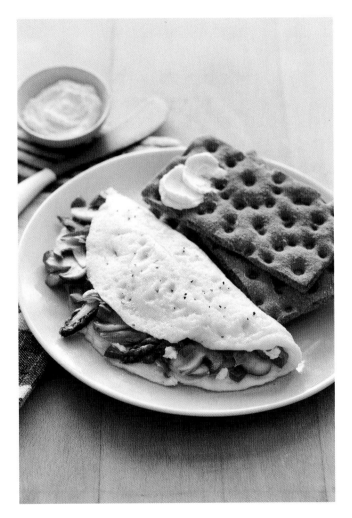

Olive oil spray

4 egg whites, beaten

2 cups chopped mixed veggies (precook, if desired)

1 teaspoon soft goat cheese, crumbled

4 basil leaves, chopped

4 whole grain crackers

1 to 2 tablespoons creamy goat cheese spread

Mist a pan with olive oil spray and place over medium heat. Pour in the egg whites and sprinkle the veggies, cheese, and basil over half of the eggs. When the eggs are set, gently fold the plain side on top of the veggie mixture and serve with a side of crackers and spread.

slim mixer

Okay, you probably don't need me to tell you about cereal mixology—you've been mixing cereals since you were five! But what I love about this particular blend is that 1½ cups dole out just 117 to 137 little calories and a big 12-gram package of fiber fun from the cereal alone.

SERVES 1

    ½ **cup Smart Bran**
    1 cup Kamut Puffs
    1 cup unsweetened vanilla almond milk
    ½ **cup berries**

    OPTIONAL
    Scrambled egg whites or ½ cup nonfat Greek yogurt on the side

Combine all the ingredients.

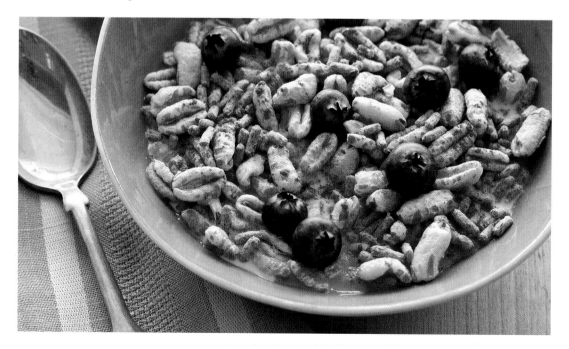

tasty mixology

This mix is the fave of my hard-to-sell patients (even college students) who dread "rabbit pellets." (I promise, Smart Bran is tastier than it looks!) What makes it great: the Sunrise offers a few different textures that change the rabbit pellet appearance. The protein, fiber, cinnamon, and dash of fruit all work together to make one tummy-filling, energy-sustaining combo. It's so good, patients often ask, "This is okay, for real?"

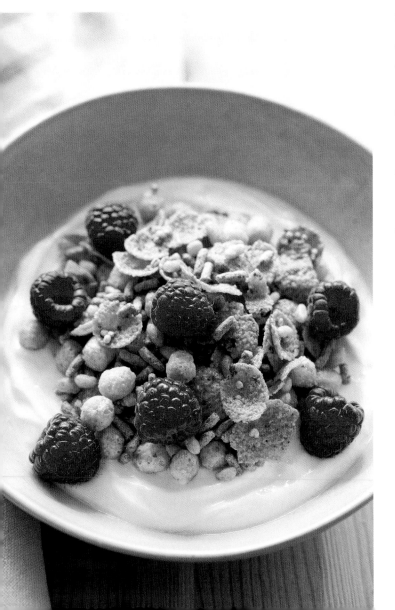

SERVES 1

½ cup **Smart Bran**
½ cup **Crunchy Maple Sunrise cereal**
6 ounces **nonfat Greek yogurt**
¼ cup **berries**

OPTIONAL
¼ teaspoon **ground cinnamon**

Combine all the ingredients.

breakfast burrito

Starting your day with a little spice will change your attitude about everything. ("Good morning, world—bring it on!") It's so easy, too.

Olive oil spray
Diced onion and bell pepper (as much as you like)
2 egg whites
½ cup cooked black beans
1 small Ezekiel tortilla or 1 large low-carb tortilla
1 pinch (½ ounce) Mexican cheese blend
Salsa

Mist a skillet with olive oil spray and heat over medium heat. Add the veggies and sauté until soft; add the egg whites and some of the beans and scramble until cooked through. Pile the mixture onto a tortilla, top with cheese and salsa, roll the whole thing up, and serve.

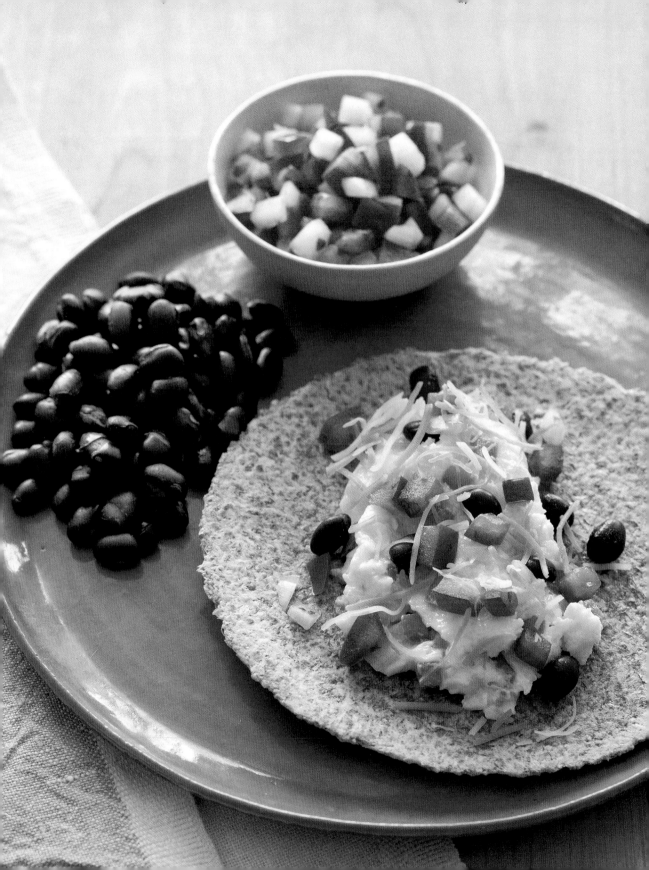

breakfast parfait options

OPTION 1 strawberry-fiber cake parfait

Okay, now you must think I'm joking around. A parfait for breakfast? Absolutely—if it's one of these!

SERVES 1

6 ounces nonfat Greek yogurt
1 Fiber Cake, crushed (page 98)
½ cup sliced strawberries
   (or a mix of berries)

Layer the yogurt in a glass with the fiber cake and strawberries and serve.

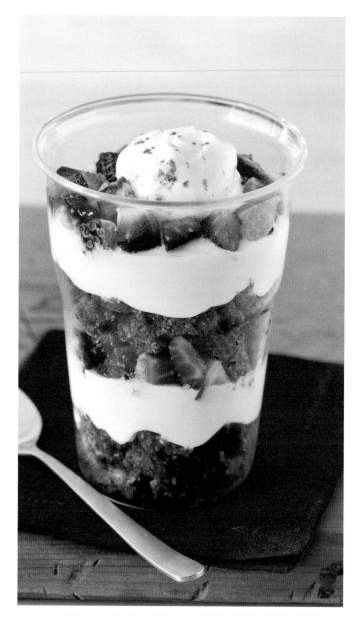

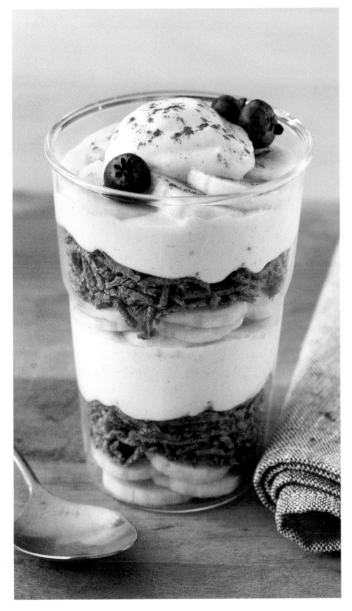

OPTION 2 honey-banana parfait

Here's another parfait that will make you think you're doing dessert for breakfast.

SERVES 1

> **6 ounces nonfat Greek yogurt**
> **1 teaspoon honey**
> **¼ teaspoon ground cinnamon**
> **½ cup All-Bran cereal**
> **1 small banana, diced**
> **Blueberries for topping**

In a bowl, stir the yogurt, honey, and cinnamon together. Layer the mixture in a glass with the cereal and banana, top with a few blueberries, and grab a spoon.

fiber cakes

I've been recommending fiber cakes (from Zen Bakery at Whole Foods Markets and at Trader Joe's under the Trader Joe's brand) for years. My patients have dubbed them "hockey pucks" because of their appearance. But the truth is they're the perfect combo of high fiber and chewy goodness. And they're so versatile: You can eat them in the morning as a cereal alternative, break them up and sprinkle them on yogurt with fruit to make a parfait, or melt dark chocolate inside them to make a chocolate lava cake (an all-time favorite; see page 74). Sounds amazing, right?

One problem: Not everyone has a Trader Joe's or Whole Foods nearby that carries them; people have begged me to come up with a recipe. So here is my version.

MAKES 9 CAKES

3½ cups wheat bran
⅓ cup whole wheat flour
2 teaspoons ground cinnamon
1 teaspoon baking powder
⅛ teaspoon salt
1 cup unsweetened organic applesauce
1 cup white grape or apple juice (preferably organic)
2 tablespoons honey (optional)
1 small apple, peeled, cored, and diced (about ¾ cup)
1 cup frozen blueberries

1. Preheat the oven to 350°F.

2. In a large bowl, mix all the dry ingredients, then add the wet ingredients and mix well with a large spoon. Fold in the diced apple. The mixture will be very thick and dense.

3. Line a muffin tin with 9 paper cups. Spoon the mixture into the cups, pressing it in as needed to fit. Press a few blueberries into each muffin.

4. Bake for 30 to 35 minutes, or until semifirm. Remove the muffins from the tin and cool them on a wire rack.

These muffins last up to a week refrigerated, and you can freeze them as well. Many people tell me that they taste better after sitting in the fridge for a day. Start baking!

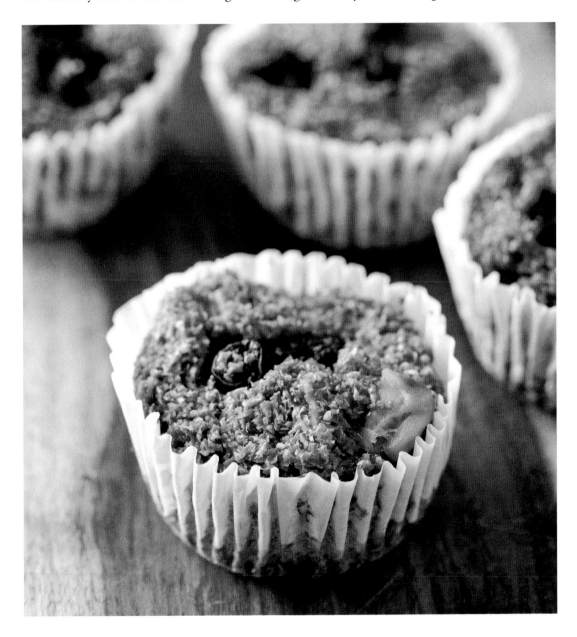

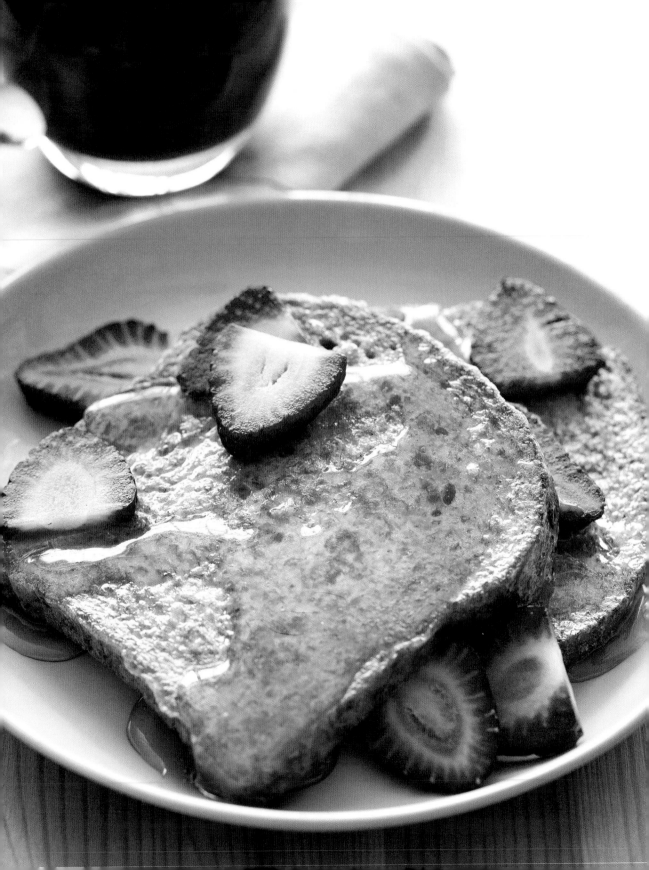

french toast the fiber way

Can French toast really be part of a nutritious breakfast? *Mais oui!* But you gotta make it like this!

SERVES 1

1 whole egg, plus 2 egg whites

2 slices whole grain bread

Olive oil spray

¼ teaspoon ground cinnamon

2 large strawberries, hulled and sliced

2 tablespoons Joseph's Sugar Free Syrup (page 199)

    or 1 teaspoon pure maple syrup

Whisk the egg with the egg whites in a wide, shallow bowl, then dip in the bread slices. Lightly coat a pan with olive oil spray and place over medium heat. Add the coated bread to the pan and cook until both sides turn golden. Top with cinnamon, berries, and syrup.

NOTE: Since brands of bread vary in fiber amount, fill in the gaps with fruit if needed.

a.m. body fuel smoothie

I know many people who just gotta have their a.m. smoothie fix for the long commute and longer hours at work or school. But skip the pricey, high-cal takeout kinds—with my breakfast smoothie, you get your fiber and protein while keeping your diet budget in check. The secret trick: hemp protein powder along with chia seeds and berries! Don't get turned off by the powder's green color—it has a smooth, nutty flavor that blends perfectly with the fruit and almond milk.

SERVES 1

1 cup unsweetened vanilla almond milk
2 tablespoons vanilla-flavored organic hemp protein powder
1 tablespoon white chia seeds
1 cup frozen blueberries
½ frozen banana

Blend all the ingredients together until smooth and serve.

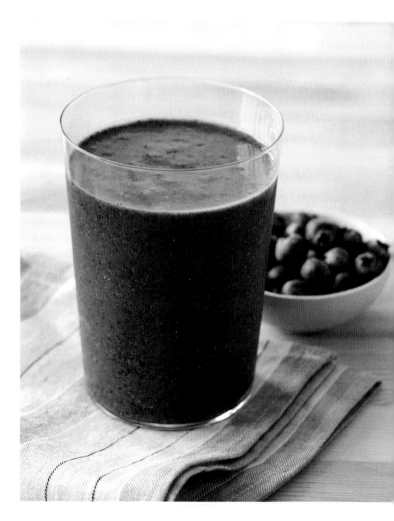

cinnamon-scented a.m. quinoa

Want a great gluten-free cereal? Here it is! Since ¾ cup of quinoa has only 3.8 grams of fiber, this calls for double boosting (just like oatmeal). Be sure to add the chia seeds and fruit to meet your fiber goal.

SERVES 1

¾ cup cooked quinoa (see Note)
1 tablespoon white chia seeds
½ cup sliced peaches or berries
Ground cinnamon
Optional: grated nutmeg or my Shaker-Waker-Upper (page 28)

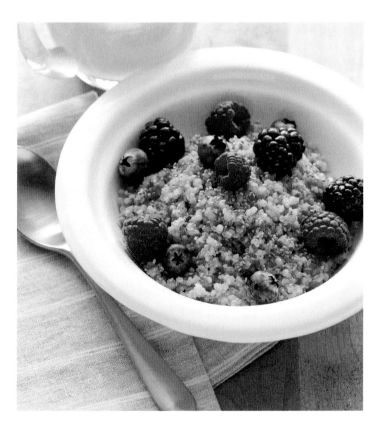

In a bowl, combine the quinoa, chia seeds, and fruit. Top with the cinnamon and nutmeg, if using.

NOTE: Cook ¼ cup raw quinoa in ½ cup unsweetened almond milk for 15 minutes to yield ¾ cup cooked quinoa. Be sure to rinse the quinoa prior to cooking.

breakfast scramble options

OPTION 1 egg and toast

Eggs are such an amazing (and affordable) source of protein. And this dish feels particularly hearty. Remember breads and crackers vary in fiber content, so enhance these recipes by adding some veg or fruit if necessary.

SERVES 1

- **2 slices whole grain bread, toasted**
- **1 Laughing Cow Light cheese wedge**
- **4 egg whites, scrambled**
- **1 large tomato, sliced**

Arrange everything on a plate and serve.

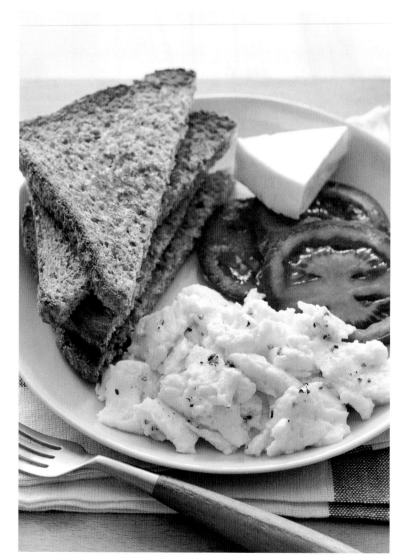

OPTION 2 egg and cracker

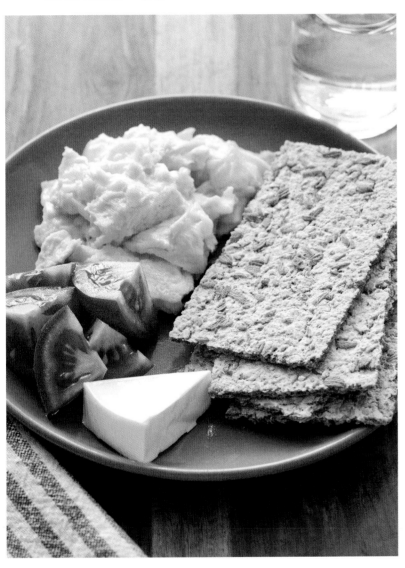

More eggs! I love the crunch crackers add to this even simpler variation (no toasting required).

SERVES 1

5 Kavli Golden Rye crispbreads (or any other fiber crispbread)
Laughing Cow Light cheese wedge or 2 tablespoons creamy goat cheese
1 whole omega-3–enriched egg plus 2 egg whites, scrambled
1 large tomato, cut into chunks

Arrange everything on a plate and serve.

double-boosted oatmeal

Fiber insurance isn't an option—it's a must if you're trying to shed some pounds and gain prevention. A cup of steel-cut oatmeal delivers only 4 grams of fiber, so you need to double boost with chia seeds and a full fruit serving. That additional 8 grams or so of fiber (for a total of 12 grams) will seal the deal!

SERVES 1

- **1 cup cooked steel-cut oatmeal**
- **1 small unpeeled apple, diced**
- **1 tablespoon white chia seeds**
- **¼ teaspoon ground cinnamon**

Warm the oatmeal, mix in the diced apple, chia seeds, and sprinkle with cinnamon.

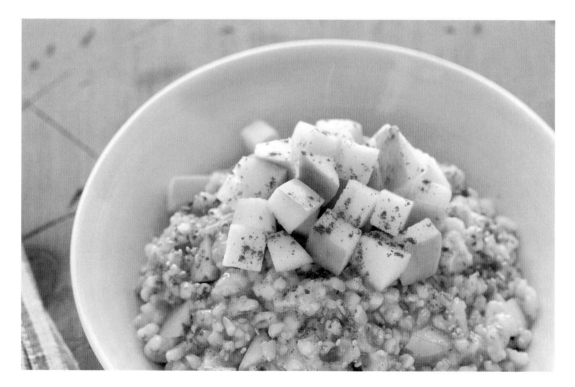

lunch

Using my Flip-It Method, you can build amazing meals! Feel free to have lunch for dinner and vice versa, and share these fun flipped menus with your friends and family—they'll be enticed to join you!

mediterranean chopped salad

SERVES 1

¾ to 1 cup canned garbanzo beans, drained and rinsed

Chopped cucumbers, tomatoes, yellow bell peppers (any amount you like)

1 to 2 tablespoons chopped fresh basil and parsley (optional)

1 to 2 teaspoons olive oil

2 tablespoons fresh lemon juice

Pinch of salt

⅓ to ⅔ cup cooled cooked quinoa on the side (optional)

Combine all the ingredients and serve.

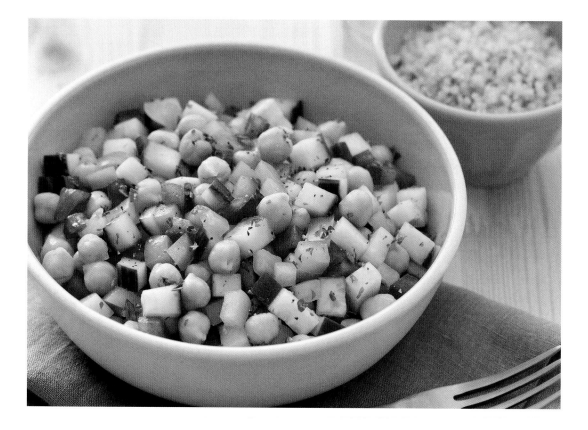

grass-fed beef burger lettuce wrap

This is a great make-at-home *or* dining-out option! Just ask your server to hold the bun and simply wrap the burger in lettuce leaves, and, of course, always swap fries for veg. (No, it's not a weird request. I see it all the time.)

SERVES 1

4-ounce lean grass-fed beef patty, cooked
2 large romaine or red-leaf lettuce leaves
Sliced pickles
Sliced tomato
1 tablespoon low-fat Thousand Island dressing (optional)

ON THE SIDE
1½ cups crudités
1 tablespoon hummus

Assemble your burger and serve with the sides.

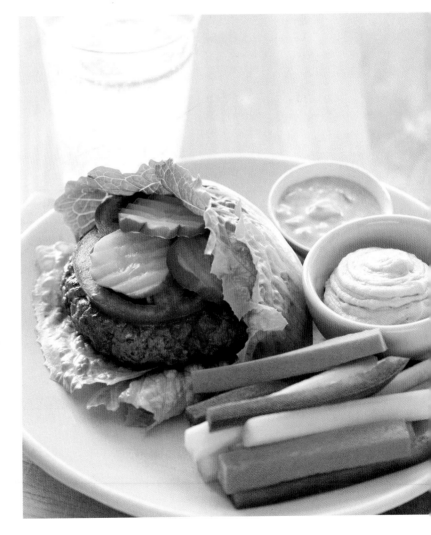

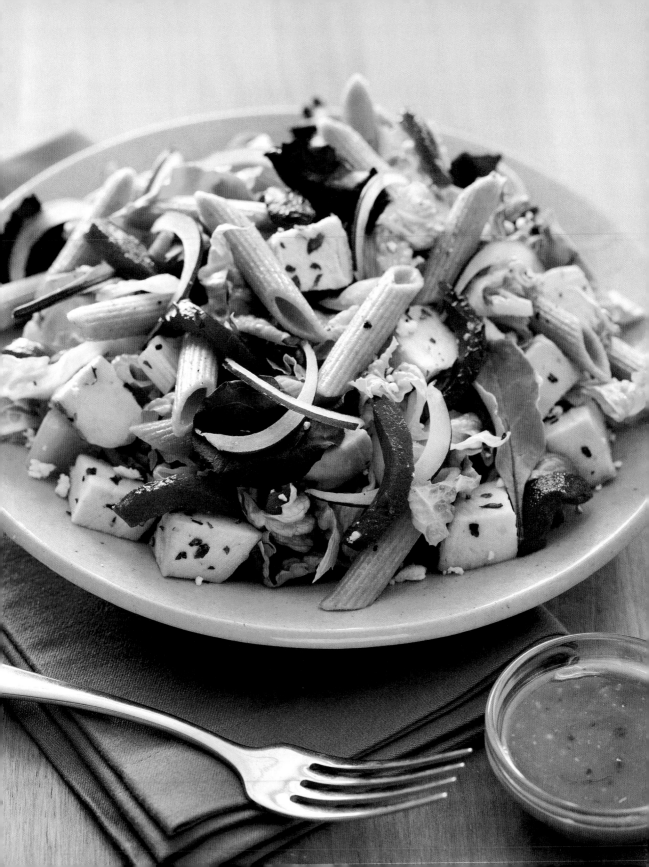

italian chicken salad

1½ to 2 cups baby arugula or mixed greens

3 to 4 ounces cooked chicken breast, cubed

½ to 1 ounce shredded mozzarella or crumbled feta cheese

2 tablespoons rinsed, sliced, jarred roasted red peppers, or jarred sun-dried
  tomatoes

½ cup cooked whole wheat pasta (optional)

Dash of dried Italian herb mix (or oregano)

1 to 2 teaspoons olive oil and 1 tablespoon balsamic vinegar, or 2 tablespoons
  of one of my recommended bottled dressings (see page 190)

Combine the greens, chicken, cheese, sun-dried tomatoes, and pasta, if using, and toss with
the herb mix. Drizzle with the dressing.

shrimp and veggie kabobs with artichoke-parmesan salad

These are great cold, too: You can do 'em ahead of time and bring them to work for lunch.

SERVES 1

3 wooden skewers
4 to 6 ounces raw shrimp, peeled and deveined
1 red or yellow pepper, cored, seeded, and cut into large squares
½ onion, cut into large squares
Salt and freshly ground black pepper
Olive oil spray
Artichoke-Parmesan Salad (recipe follows)

Soak the skewers in water for 10 minutes or so to prevent burning. Thread the shrimp, pepper, and onion alternately on the skewers and season with salt and pepper. Mist a grill pan with olive oil spray and grill the kabobs over medium heat, turning once, just until the shrimp turn pink and are cooked through (3 to 5 minutes, depending on the size of the shrimp). Serve the kabobs with the artichoke-Parmesan salad on the side.

artichoke-parmesan salad

SERVES 1

1 cup mixed greens
4 jarred or canned artichoke hearts, rinsed
2 tablespoons shaved Parmesan cheese
2 tablespoons low-cal balsamic vinaigrette

Combine all the ingredients in a small bowl and serve with the kabobs.

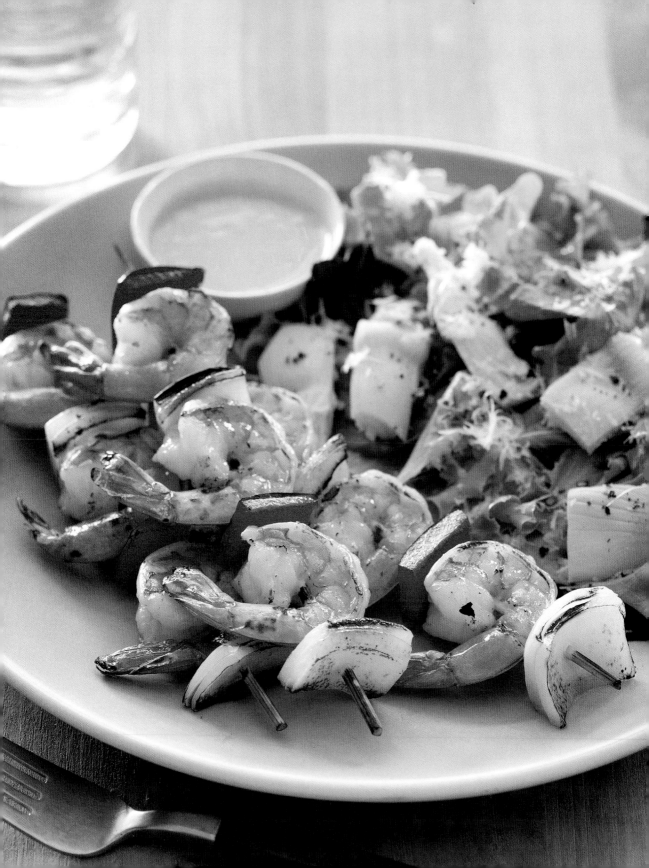

hearty lentil soup

This is an all-inclusive vegetable-and-protein soup. I like to freeze individual servings (1½ cups) and keep them at work. It's also an easy meal to approximate when eating out! Go for a large bowl of brothy lentil soup, and add a side salad or any steamed veg, plus half a pita, if you like.

SERVES 6 TO 8

- **1 tablespoon olive oil**
- **1 small onion, chopped**
- **2 carrots, peeled and thinly sliced**
- **2 celery stalks, chopped**
- **3 garlic cloves, minced**
- **2 cups dried petite lentils**
- **2 Roma tomatoes, chopped**
- **1 tablespoon tomato paste**
- **2 large zucchini, sliced and quartered**
- **2 cups chopped Swiss chard or spinach**
- **8 cups low-sodium chicken or vegetable broth, plus more if needed**
- **1 bay leaf**
- **¼ teaspoon dried thyme**
- **¼ teaspoon kosher salt**
- **¼ teaspoon ground black pepper**

Heat the olive oil in a large pot over medium heat. Add the onion, carrots, celery, and garlic, and sauté for 2 minutes. Reduce the heat to low and cook for 5 minutes, or until tender. Add the lentils, stir to combine, and cook for another 3 minutes. Increase the heat to medium, add the tomatoes, tomato paste, zucchini, Swiss chard, broth, and bay leaf and bring to a boil. Reduce the heat to low again and simmer until the lentils are tender, 25 to 30 minutes. Add the thyme, salt, and black pepper. Add more broth, if needed, to thin the soup out. Remove the bay leaf and serve.

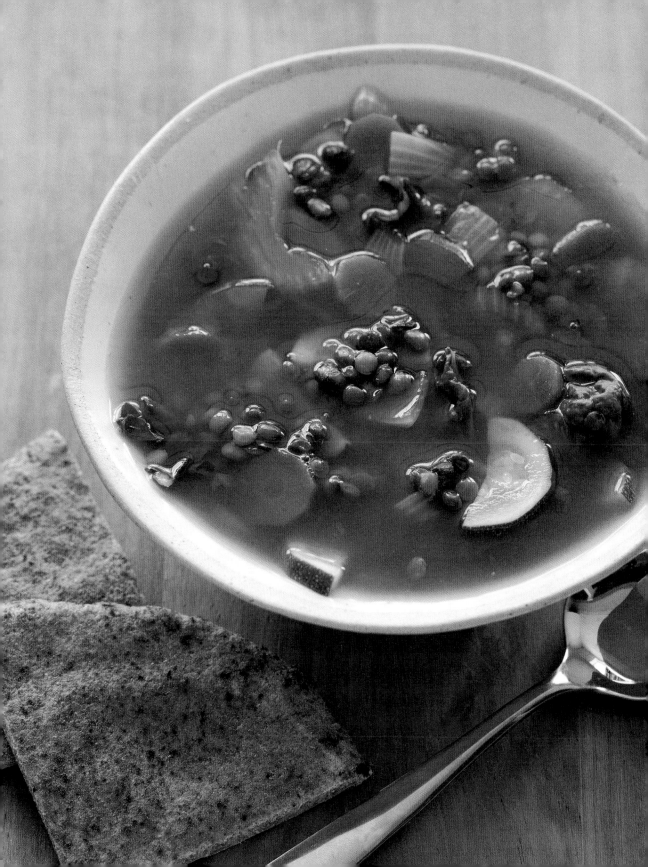

stuffed tomatoes
with garlic asparagus

Olive oil spray

2 beefsteak tomatoes, cored and partially hollowed out

¾ cup Sunday Salad made with tuna (page 47)

½ to 1 ounce grated part-skim mozzarella cheese

8 to 10 asparagus spears, tough ends snapped off

Garlic salt to taste

1 or 2 Wasa crackers (optional)

Preheat the oven to 375°F. Mist a rimmed baking sheet with olive oil spray. Stuff half of the tuna salad into each tomato, place them on the sheet, and top with the cheese. Lay the asparagus on the sheet alongside, lightly mist them with olive oil spray. Season with a touch of garlic salt. Bake until the cheese melts and the asparagus is tender but still crisp, 5 to 10 minutes. Serve with the crackers if you like.

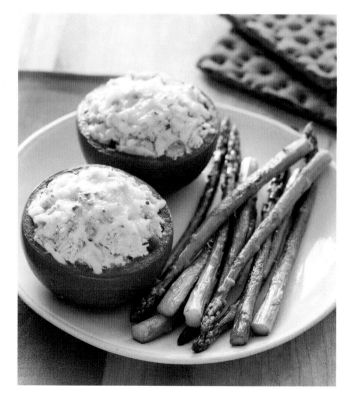

salmon hand rolls

Shout out: This looks fancy, but it's *super* simple—you can throw it together in less than a minute, since you're using one of your premade Sunday Salads.

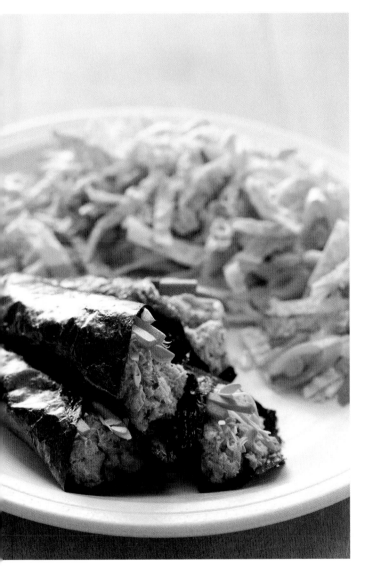

½ **cup to ¾ cup Sunday Salad**
    made with salmon (page 47)
3 to 4 nori seaweed sheets
Julienne-cut carrots
Sprouts
1 tablespoon light dressing
Side salad (with any dark greens or
    cabbage you have on hand)

Place a scoop of salmon salad on each seaweed sheet, sprinkle the carrots and sprouts on top, add the dressing, roll up, and serve with a side salad.

soup-and-sandwich combo

SERVES 1

MAKE AN OPEN-FACED SANDWICH:

1 slice high-fiber whole grain bread
½ cup Egg White-*ish* salad (page 53)
1 lettuce leaf
2 to 3 tomato slices
Dash of paprika

SERVE WITH:

1 to 1½ cups Ultimate Low-Cal
Veggie Soup (recipe opposite)

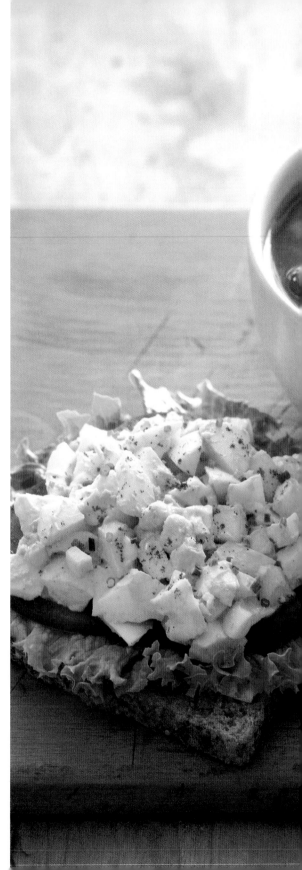

ultimate low-cal veggie soup

Olive oil spray
3 celery stalks, chopped
1 large carrot, chopped
1 cup diced yellow onion
2 garlic cloves, minced
One 28-ounce can or Tetra Pak
    crushed tomatoes
8 cups low-sodium vegetable broth
2 tablespoons tomato paste
2 medium zucchini, sliced
1 cup green beans, cut in half
3 cups chopped green or Chinese
    cabbage
1 tablespoon dried Italian herb mix

Mist a large pot with olive oil spray and heat it over medium heat. Add the celery, carrot, onion, and garlic and sauté for 5 to 7 minutes, until just tender. Add the crushed tomatoes and vegetable broth. Bring to a boil, then add the tomato paste, zucchini, green beans, and cabbage. Bring the soup to a boil again, then cover, reduce the heat to low, and simmer until the vegetables are tender, 15 to 20 minutes. Add the herb mix.

penne and meatballs

Refrigerate the leftover meatballs and sauce for a quick-fix dinner or lunch later in the week. They also freeze well.

SERVES 1

1½ cups broccoli florets, steamed
½ cup cooked whole wheat penne
3 or 4 Turkey Meatballs with ½ cup sauce (recipe follows)
1 tablespoon grated Parmesan cheese

Combine the broccoli, penne, and meatballs with their sauce. Sprinkle with the Parmesan and serve.

turkey meatballs

MAKES 10 TO 12 MEATBALLS (SERVES 3 TO 4)

1 pound 99 percent fat-free ground turkey
½ cup cooked quinoa
1 egg, lightly beaten
1 tablespoon fresh oregano or 1 teaspoon dried
1 teaspoon dried thyme
¼ to ½ teaspoon kosher salt, to taste
½ cup minced onion
2 garlic cloves, minced
Olive oil spray
Two 24-ounce jars low-sodium marinara sauce

1. In a large bowl, combine the turkey, quinoa, egg, oregano, thyme, and salt. Coat a skillet with olive oil spray, place it over medium-low heat, and sauté the onion and garlic until translucent, 2 to 4 minutes. Cool. Combine the onion and garlic with the turkey mixture.

2. Roll the mixture into 2-inch meatballs. Pour the marinara sauce into a large pot and gently add the meatballs. Turn the heat to medium, cover, and bring to a simmer, then reduce the heat to medium-low and cook for 20 minutes, or until the meatballs are cooked through.

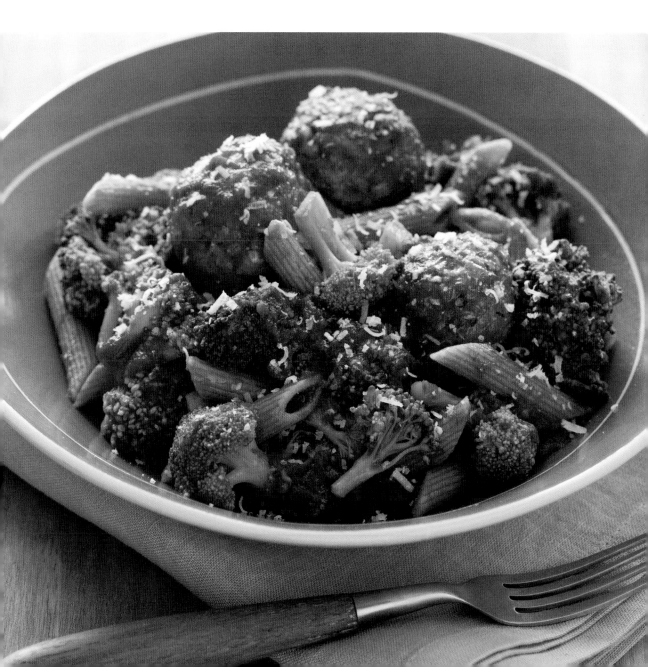

OUT TO LUNCH niçoise salad

Seared tuna steak

Hard-boiled egg

Green beans

Tomato wedges

Niçoise olives

Anchovy fillets (optional)

Small red new potatoes (optional)

Balsamic or lemon vinaigrette

ORDERING ADVICE: Ask for the dressing on the side (always), and eat no more than 1 egg yolk. Feel free to ask them to hold the potatoes if you're not doing carbs.

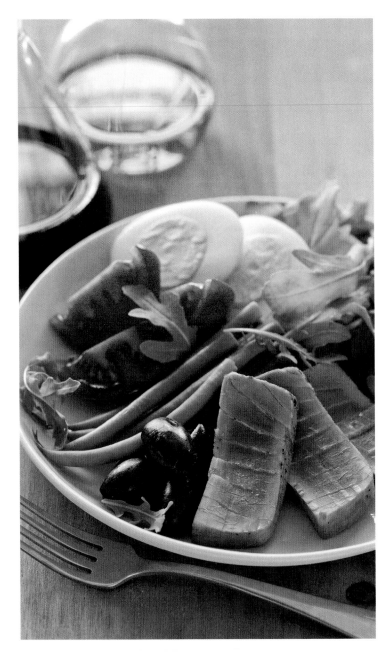

dinner

Most people like to save the best for last, and these dinner ideas make the perfect way to top your day. Can't wait? Then don't! You can have these dinner recipes for lunch since the calorie portions are the same. And if you like them so much, you can have them again!

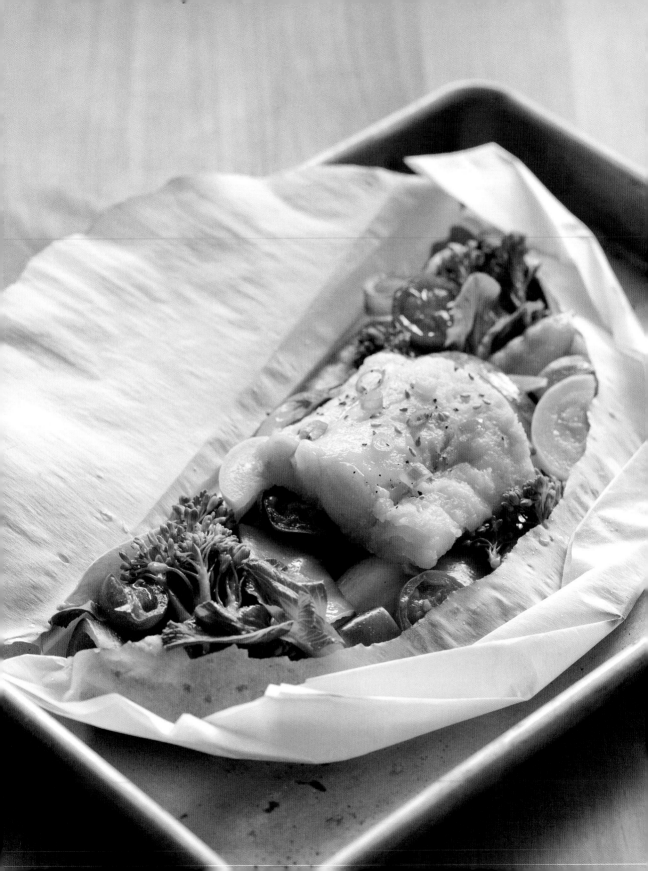

one-shot-deal dinner

Simply toss your protein and veggies into parchment paper, seal, bake—and you're good to go. No cleanup!

SERVES 1

2 cups any veggies, cut into bite-size pieces
½ **garlic clove, minced**
Salt and freshly ground black pepper
4 ounces black cod fillet
½ **teaspoon reduced-sodium soy sauce or Bragg Liquid Aminos (page 195)**
1 scallion, white and light green parts, thinly sliced
¼ **cup vegetable broth**
Splash of dry white wine
Sesame seeds
Lemon wedges

Preheat the oven to 375°F. Lay a big rectangle of parchment paper on a baking sheet; place the veggies and minced garlic on one end of the paper and season lightly with salt and pepper. Place the fish on top of the veggies and brush with the soy sauce. Add the scallion. Sprinkle the vegetable broth and a splash of white wine over the whole thing. Fold the parchment over the fish and veggies and, beginning at one end, crimp the edges to seal it completely (you'll wind up with a semicircle-shaped packet). Bake for 10 to 15 minutes, then set aside to cool for 5 minutes. Open the parchment, sprinkle the fish with sesame seeds, add a squeeze of lemon juice, and serve.

tofu ratatouille

Think you don't like tofu? Guaranteed this meal will change your mind! The tofu absorbs loads of flavor from all the spices and tomato sauce. A must try.

SERVES 4

Olive oil spray
1 cup sliced carrots
1 small onion, chopped
¼ cup chopped fresh basil
2 teaspoons chopped fresh thyme
2 teaspoons minced garlic (about 4 cloves)
2 cups diced eggplant
2 cups diced zucchini
2 cups chopped tomatoes
Two 14-ounce cans or Tetra Paks no-salt-added tomato sauce
2 cups (one 14-ounce package) firm organic tofu, drained and chopped
1 teaspoon ground cumin
½ teaspoon salt
⅛ teaspoon freshly ground black pepper
One 8-ounce bag Shirataki Noodles (page 171), rinsed (optional)

Mist a large sauté pan with olive oil spray and place it over medium-high heat. Add the carrots and sauté for 4 minutes, then toss in the onion, basil, thyme, and garlic and cook 4 minutes more. Add the eggplant and zucchini and sauté for 4 minutes. Stir in the tomatoes and tomato sauce and bring to a boil. Add the tofu cubes, reduce the heat to medium-low, and simmer for 30 minutes, gently stirring occasionally. Remove from the heat and stir in the cumin, salt, pepper, and noodles, if using.

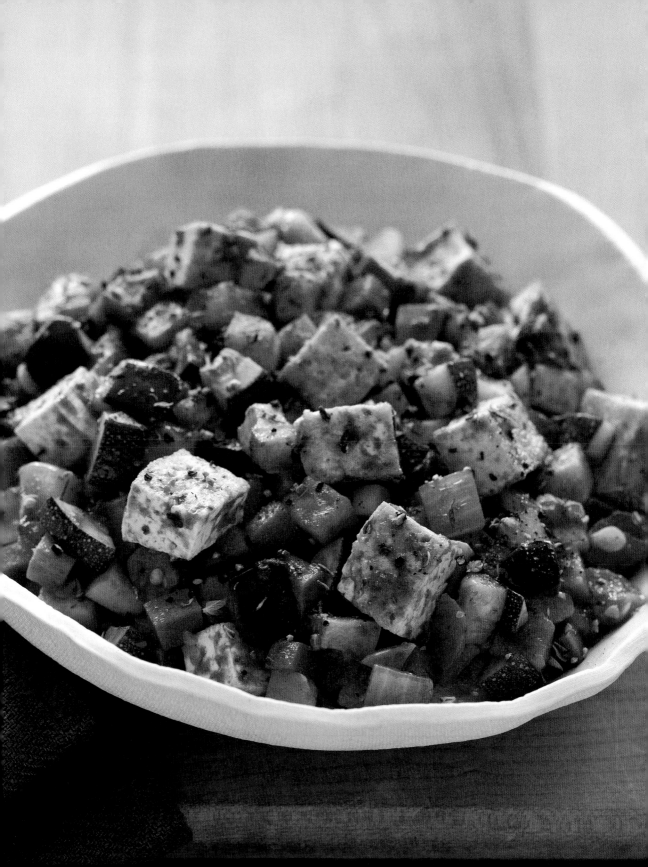

glazed teriyaki salmon with zucchini and cauliflower mash

SERVES 1

2 tablespoons reduced-sodium teriyaki sauce
One 4- to 6-ounce wild salmon fillet
Olive oil spray
½ teaspoon olive oil
2 small zucchini or squash, thinly sliced
½ cup sliced mushrooms (any kind you like)
1 scallion, white and light green parts, chopped
½ teaspoon toasted sesame seeds
1 serving Cauliflower Mash (recipe follows)

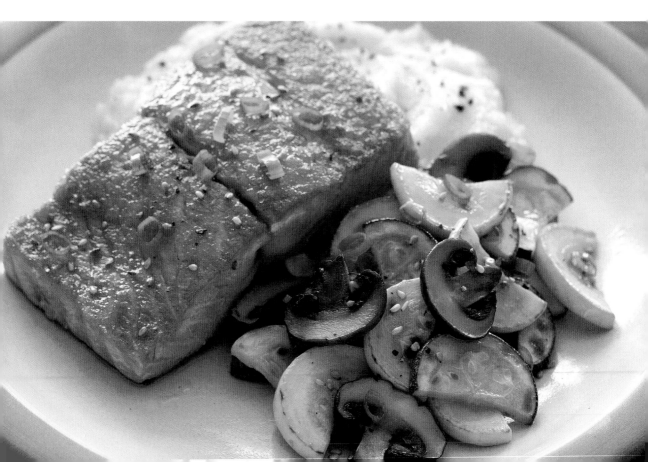

1. Place the teriyaki sauce and fish in a resealable plastic bag and marinate in the fridge for 20 minutes. Remove the fish and discard the marinade.

2. Heat the skillet over medium-low heat and lightly coat with olive oil spray. Add the salmon and sear it for 5 minutes, then flip it and sear the other side for 5 minutes, or until the fish is cooked to your liking. Set the salmon aside on a plate and cover to keep warm.

3. Add the olive oil, zucchini, mushrooms, and scallion to the same skillet and sauté until lightly browned, about 4 minutes. Sprinkle with the sesame seeds and serve with the salmon.

cauliflower mash

SERVES 3

Olive oil spray
1 small onion, chopped
1 large head cauliflower, chopped
1 garlic clove, minced
6 cups low-sodium vegetable broth
Salt and freshly ground black pepper

Mist the bottom of a medium pot with olive oil spray and place it over medium heat. Add the onion and sauté for 2 minutes, then reduce the heat to low, cover the pot, and sweat the onion for 5 to 7 minutes (do not brown). Add the cauliflower, garlic, and just enough broth to cover the cauliflower and cook, covered, for 30 minutes, or until the cauliflower is very tender. Use a slotted spoon to remove the veggies to a blender and puree or use an immersion blender. (Discard the broth or use it for soup.) Puree until smooth, then add salt and pepper to taste.

TIP: This recipe serves 3 since everyone wants leftovers of this creamy veg dish. Feel free to double or triple the recipe. You can also simply toss a bunch of veg in the remaining broth and you have yourself a quick and easy low-cal soup.

veggie fajita

SERVES 1

PICK UP FROM A MEXICAN JOINT:

¾ **cup black beans (from a 1-quart container)**

2 cups fajita veggie mix (sautéed sliced bell peppers, onions, and mushrooms)

One 6-inch corn tortilla (optional)

Pico de gallo

½ **to 1 ounce shredded Mexican cheese**

Hot sauce to taste

ORDERING ADVICE: Be sure to ask for the veggies "easy on the oil" to avoid a grease-trap scenario. This meal is also simple to DIY at home—just roast strips of peppers and onions on a baking sheet, open a can of black beans (be sure to rinse them), add salsa and ½ to 1 ounce of grated cheese, and you're good to go!

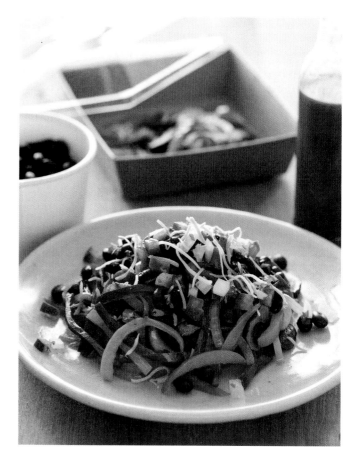

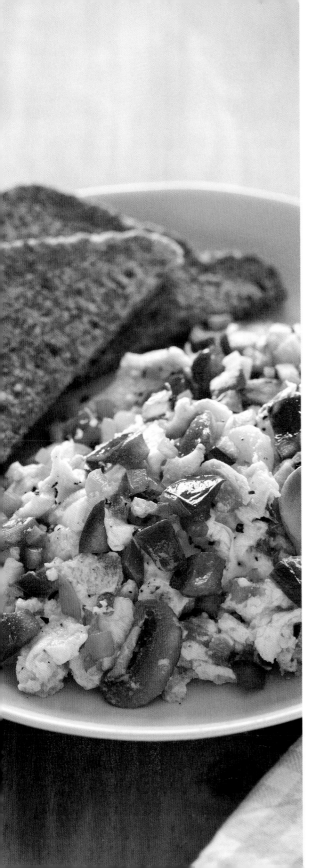

breakfast for dinner—fast!

This is what I whip up when I come home late and my inner voice is yelling, "I gotta eat!" Should I pick up the phone or save time and money? No question: This "starter kit" meal can be on a plate in less than five minutes.

SERVES 1

Olive oil spray
1 garlic clove, minced
1 large tomato, diced
3 to 4 mushrooms, sliced
½ green bell pepper, cored, seeded,
    and chopped
Any other veg you like
Pinch of salt and freshly ground
    black pepper
1 whole egg plus 4 egg whites, beaten
1 slice whole grain bread, toasted (optional)

Lightly coat a skillet with olive oil and heat it over medium heat. Add the garlic, tomato, mushrooms, pepper, and any other desired veggies and sauté for 2 to 3 minutes, until softened. Season lightly with salt and pepper, add the eggs, and scramble away! Serve with the toast, if desired.

bbq chicken with crunchy coleslaw

Crunchy, creamy coleslaw, really? Absolutely—if it's my lightened-up version. Dig in!

SERVES 1

4 to 6 ounces grilled chicken breast

1 tablespoon low-sugar BBQ sauce (to brush on chicken or for dunking)

1½ cups Crunchy Coleslaw (recipe follows)

crunchy coleslaw

SERVES 4 TO 6

5 tablespoons plain nonfat Greek yogurt

2 tablespoons reduced-fat Vegenaise or reduced-fat mayonnaise

1½ tablespoons fresh lemon juice

1½ teaspoons spicy Dijon mustard

1½ cups shredded red cabbage

1½ cups shredded green cabbage (Savoy works well)

½ cup shredded carrots

1 scallion, white and light green parts, thinly sliced

½ cup shredded fennel or grated jicama (optional)

Pinch of salt and freshly ground black pepper

Whisk the yogurt, Vegenaise, lemon juice, and mustard together in a large bowl. Add the veggies and toss together until well mixed; season with salt and pepper. It's best to marinate it for at least an hour before serving. Store leftovers. It keeps for a couple of days in the fridge.

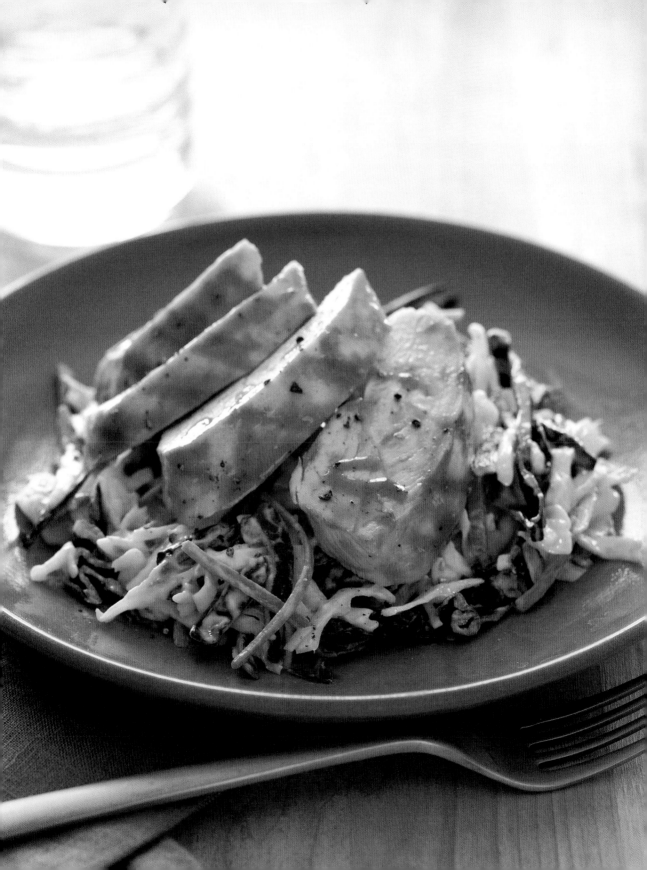

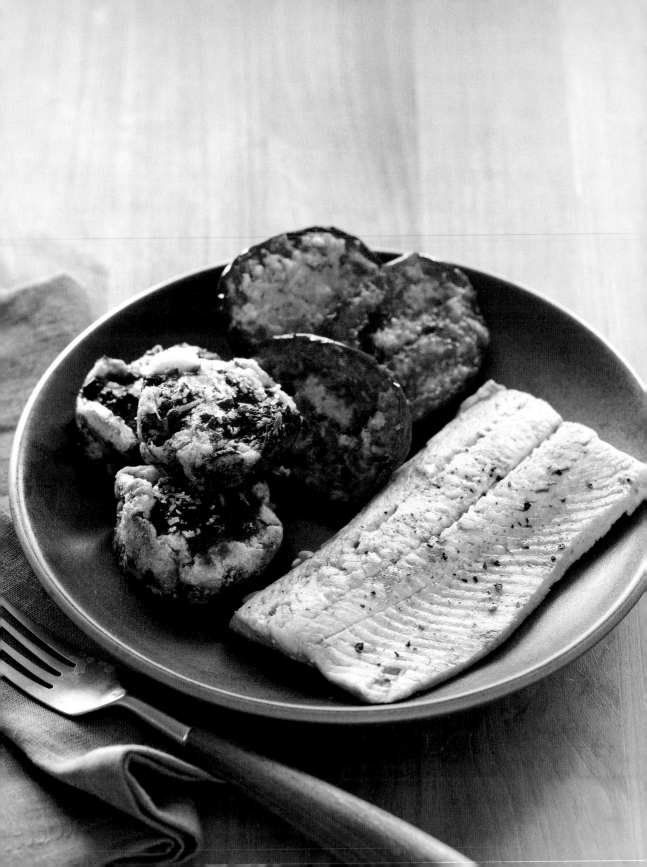

broiled trout with mini spinach soufflés and parm tomatoes

This is a starter-kit recipe that I give to every patient—it's done in minutes, and once you plate the trout all you have to do is toss the foil. No pans to scrub!

SERVES 1

1 teaspoon grated Parmesan cheese
1 to 2 Roma tomatoes, halved
½ medium baked yam (optional)
1 serving Broiled Trout (recipe follows)
2 Mini Spinach Soufflés (recipe follows)

Sprinkle the cheese over the tomato halves and broil in a toaster oven until the cheese just starts to brown. Serve alongside the trout and soufflés. (You can also broil the tomatoes in the dish with the fish.)

broiled trout

SERVES 1

1 teaspoon olive oil
1 lemon
½ teaspoon Magical Mystery Mix (page 40)
¼ teaspoon paprika
One 5- to 6-ounce trout fillet

Preheat the broiler. Combine the olive oil, a squeeze of lemon juice, and the seasonings on a plate. Brush the fish with the spice mixture. Place the fish, skin side down, on a foil-lined baking sheet and broil for 5 to 7 minutes, until flaky and cooked through. Plate the fish and squeeze more lemon juice on top.

mini spinach soufflés

Consider this a veg dish with a hit of protein. A deliciously un-boring way to get your veggies in!

Olive oil spray
Two 10-ounces packages frozen spinach, thawed and
    squeezed of excess liquid
1½ cups diced mushrooms
1 garlic clove, minced
¼ cup grated Parmesan cheese, plus more for sprinkling
1 teaspoon dried oregano
10 egg whites (fresh, not from a carton)
½ cup low-sodium marinara sauce

1. Preheat the oven to 350°F and coat a muffin tin with olive oil spray.

2. In a large bowl, combine the spinach, mushrooms, garlic, Parmesan, and oregano. Mix well with a spoon.

3. In a separate bowl, use a hand or stand mixer to whip the egg whites on high speed until soft peaks form, 4 to 5 minutes. Pour the eggs over the veggies and gently fold to combine. Spoon the mixture evenly into the prepared muffin tin. Bake for 20 minutes, or until a knife inserted into the center of a soufflé comes out clean. Set the muffin tin on a rack to cool slightly before removing the soufflés. To serve, top each soufflé with a spoonful of marinara sauce and a pinch of Parmesan cheese. Serve warm.

TIP: Instead of a muffin tin, you can bake a single soufflé in a large square Pyrex dish for 25 minutes, then cut it into squares.

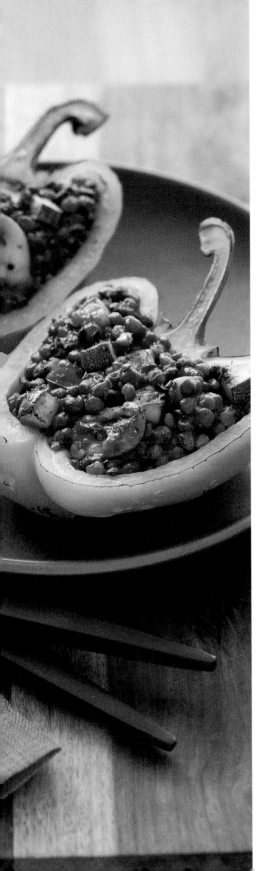

stuffed bell pepper

SERVES 1

Olive oil spray
1 cup diced zucchini
1 cup diced tomatoes
½ cup sliced mushrooms
3 tablespoons low-sodium marinara sauce
1 cup cooked lentils (simmer ½ cup uncooked lentils
**   in 1½ cups broth for about 20 minutes)**
Pinch of garlic powder
Pinch of salt
1 large bell pepper, cored, seeded, and halved
**   lengthwise**
1 teaspoon chopped fresh cilantro or parsley
**   (optional)**

1. Preheat the oven to 375°F.

2. Coat a skillet with olive oil spray and heat over medium heat. Add the zucchini, tomatoes, mushrooms, and marinara sauce and cook until the veggies are soft, about 5 minutes. Remove from the heat and stir in the lentils, garlic powder, and salt.

3. Stuff each pepper half with the lentil mixture, place the pepper halves on a baking sheet, and bake for 15 to 20 minutes, until the pepper is tender. Remove from the oven and garnish with the fresh herbs, if using.

easy chicken stir-fry

1 teaspoon minced scallion

2 teaspoons rice wine vinegar

1 teaspoon reduced-sodium soy sauce or Bragg Liquid Aminos

1 teaspoon minced peeled fresh or jarred ginger

1½ teaspoons prepared hoisin sauce

Olive oil spray

4 to 6 ounces chicken breast, cut into small strips

½ cup halved baby carrots

1 cup broccoli florets

¼ cup canned sliced water chestnuts, drained

¼ cup snow peas

½ cup sliced mushrooms

¼ cup canned bamboo shoots, drained

1. In a small bowl, combine the scallion, vinegar, soy sauce, ginger, and hoisin sauce. Set aside.

2. Mist a wok or sauté pan with olive oil spray and place it over high heat. Add the chicken and stir-fry until cooked through, 5 to 7 minutes. Remove to a bowl. Throw the carrots, broccoli, and hoisin mixture into the pan and stir-fry until the veggies are cooked but still crunchy, about 5 minutes. Add the water chestnuts, snow peas, mushrooms, bamboo shoots, and cooked chicken and stir to combine; cook for 1 to 2 minutes to heat through. Serve hot.

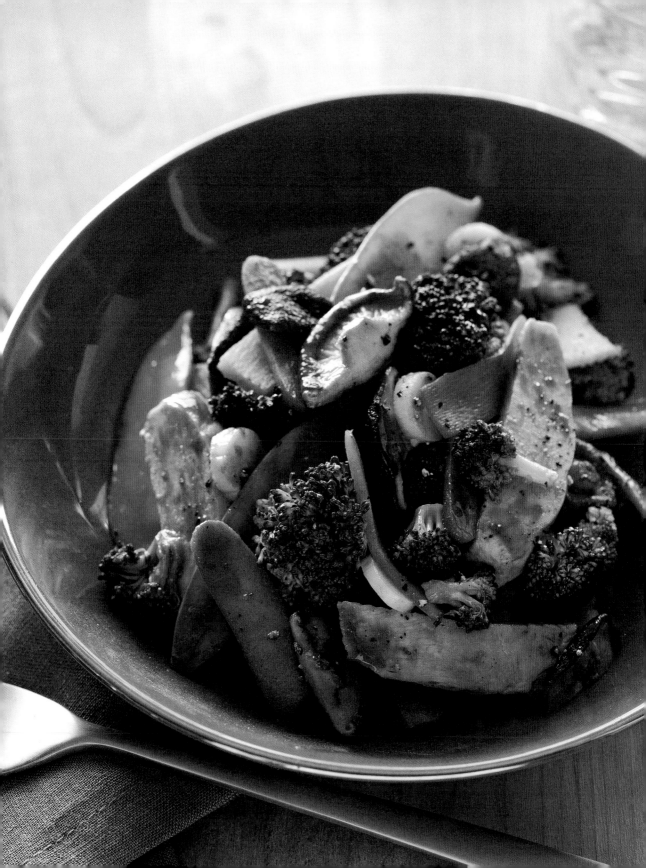

OUT TO DINNER rachel's go-to
italian dinner out!

Grilled whitefish, "easy on the oil" (try the branzino—it's my fave!)
Side of steamed spinach (not sautéed!—major calorie saver)
Side of marinara sauce
Grated Parmesan cheese

ORDERING ADVICE: I top the spinach with marinara sauce, add a sprinkle of Parmesan—and everyone's eating off my plate!

Not only am I getting great omega-3s from the fish—I've got the veg, a shot of lycopene from the marinara, and the *mmm* flavor of the Parm. Since the meal was set up right, I can enjoy a glass of wine or share a light appetizer with my date.

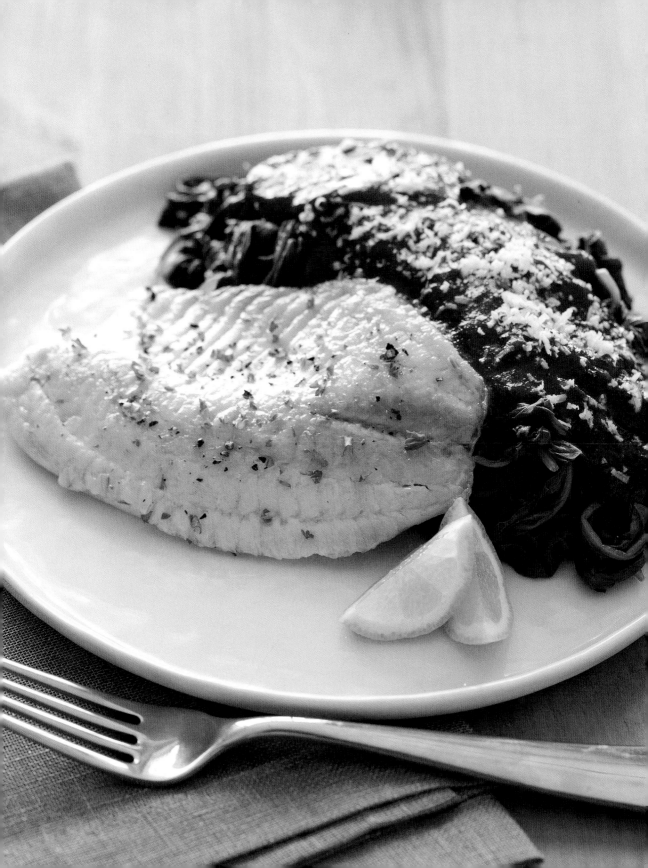

7 more ways to make seriously delicious veggies

This is one thing people always struggle with at first—seeing beyond salads and finding other creative ways to prepare produce. So I'm gonna make it easy for you!

1. make my simple broccoli soup

It's a great side dish!

- **2 teaspoons olive oil**
- **1 cup chopped yellow onion**
- **2 garlic cloves, chopped**
- **6 cups low-sodium broth (chicken or vegetable)**
- **8 cups broccoli florets**
- **¼ teaspoon black pepper**
- **Salt**

Heat the oil in a large pot over medium heat. Add the onion, reduce the heat to low, cover the pot, and sweat the onion for 5 to 7 minutes, until softened but not browned. Add the garlic, broth, and broccoli, bring to a boil, and cook for 30 minutes. Remove from the heat, add the pepper, and season with salt. Puree until smooth using an immersion blender.

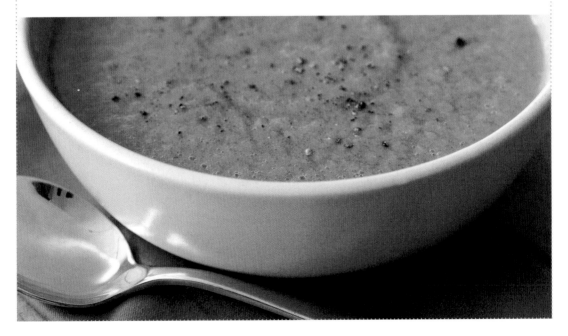

2. whip up a batch of eggplant tomato stew

Serve this in a shallow bowl with some Turkey Meatballs (page 120), sliced chicken breast, lentils, or any other protein on top.

Olive oil spray
10 Roma tomatoes, quartered
4 small eggplants (Japanese or Italian), cut into cubes
1 large garlic clove, minced
2 teaspoons dried Italian seasoning
Pinch of salt and freshly ground black pepper

Preheat the oven to 375°F. Mist a roasting pan with olive oil spray, toss in the tomatoes, eggplant, garlic, and Italian seasoning, and mist the veggies, too. Cover the pan with foil and bake for 15 minutes. Remove the foil, stir, and bake for 20 to 45 minutes, uncovered (the longer it bakes, the heartier and more stewlike it becomes). Stir well to break up the veggies and season with a pinch of salt and pepper.

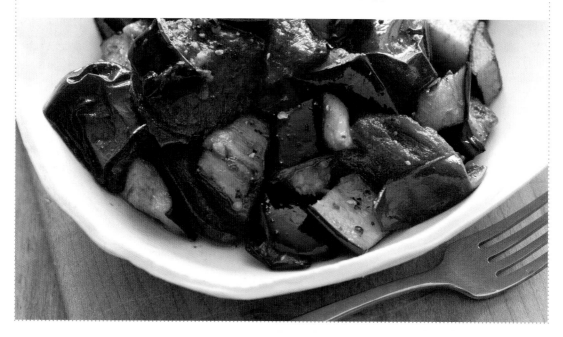

3. how about a refreshing fennel salad?

SERVES 4 TO 6

**2 large fennel bulbs, cored (discard the green stalks, but keep some of
the fronds)**
3 tablespoons fresh lemon juice
1 tablespoon extra virgin olive oil
¼ teaspoon salt

Halve each fennel bulb, then slice it into thin strips. Place the fennel in a lidded glass container with the remaining ingredients, including the fronds, put the top on, and shake to combine. Let marinate for at least 1 hour before serving.

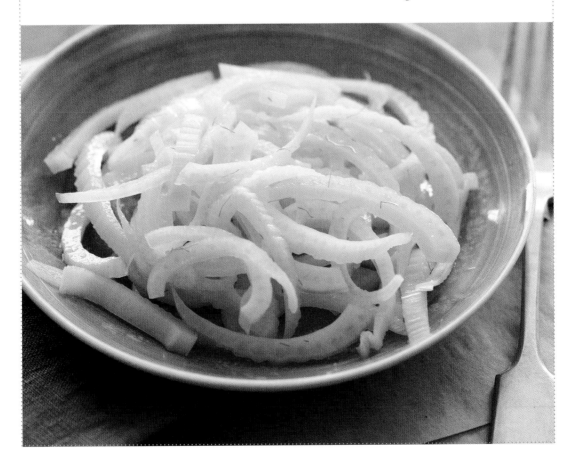

4. make my famous zucchini "spaghetti"

SERVES 2

Topped with marinara sauce and a splash of Parmesan cheese, this "mock spaghetti" is favored by many. You can prep and enjoy it as is or do a 50/50 split with whole wheat pasta, which is popular with teens.

> **2 teaspoons olive oil**
> **1 garlic clove, minced**
> **3 medium zucchini, julienned**
> **2 yellow crookneck squash, julienned**
> **½ cup low-sodium marinara sauce**
> **Dash of freshly grated Parmesan cheese**

Heat the olive oil in a sauté pan over medium heat. Add the garlic, zucchini, and squash and cook for 3 to 4 minutes, until the vegetables soften but aren't mushy. Top with the marinara sauce to taste and the Parmesan cheese.

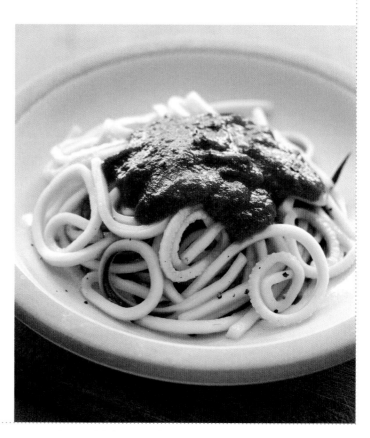

5. broccoli slaw, anyone?

SERVES 4 TO 6

This is creamy and crunchy all in one! Eat it on its own or add a few tablespoons to your mixed green salads to jazz them up in a big way.

> **1 bag shredded broccoli slaw mix**
> **½ cup low-fat, low-sodium salad dressing (I like Galeos and Bolthouse Farms yogurt-based dressings)**

Combine the slaw and dressing in a bowl, stir well, and refrigerate in a container for a few hours to overnight for the flavors to meld.

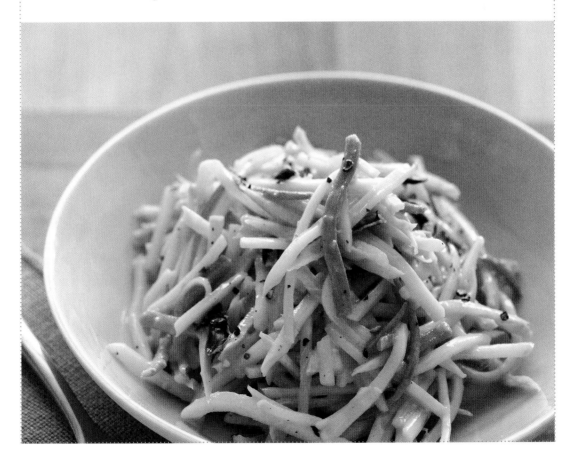

6. love this cauliflower "couscous"!

SERVES 4

A total treat since it's fluffy and tastes like the real deal.

1 head cauliflower, roughly chopped
Olive oil spray
Himalayan or kosher salt
Freshly ground black pepper
Ground turmeric

Preheat the oven to 350°F. Place the chopped cauliflower in a food processor and pulse until small, couscous-size pieces form. Dump the cauliflower onto a large cookie sheet, coat with olive oil spray and sprinkle with salt, pepper, and turmeric to taste. Roast until the cauliflower starts to turn golden brown, about 10 minutes. Stir gently and roast for 5 to 10 minutes more, until done to your liking.

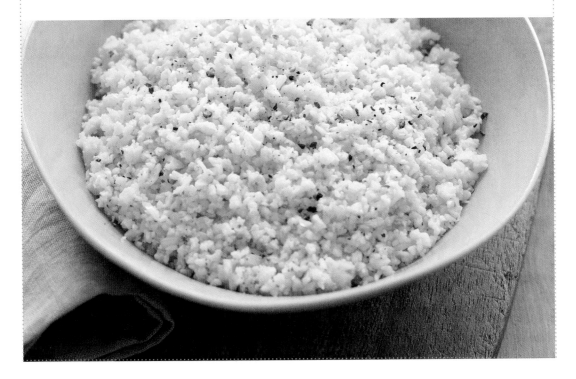

7. pesto cauliflower

SERVES 1 TO 2

Here's another way to dress up cauliflower. Pesto is great on other kinds of steamed veg as well.

2 teaspoons prepared pesto
2 cups cauliflower florets, steamed but still crunchy

Gently fold the pesto into the warm cooked cauliflower.

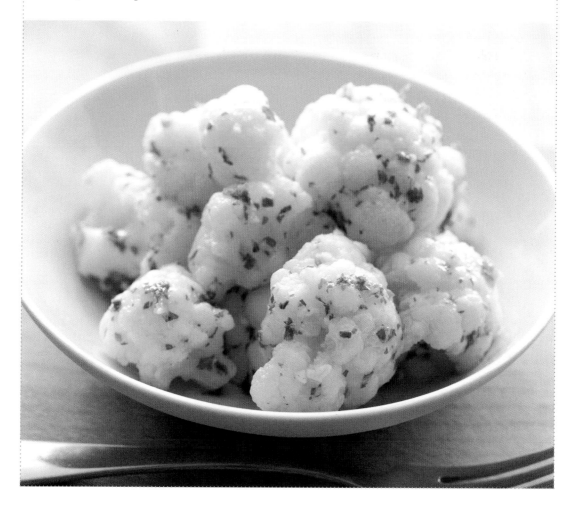

NOW *THAT'S* THE WAY YOU DINE OUT!

There's only so long most of us can stand cooking, even if the recipes taste great. Plus, we absolutely need to treat ourselves now and then. So don't feel guilty about dining out—just remember these four tips to make sure you're dining smart:

1. **KNOW BEFORE YOU GO.** If you know where you're eating before you leave home or work, try to find the restaurant's menu online (Yelp.com lists restaurants in most big cities). Now you can take your time to pick what you want, without pressure from friends, waiters, or hunger pangs. At the table you can order with confidence—and even give advice to others.

2. **JUMP TO THE VEGGIES IN THE MENU.** Restaurants don't write their menus in Flip-It-ese—they put the more profitable items where your eyes are more likely to fall. That usually means proteins. So train yourself to seek out the veg first, then build from there.

3. **ASK FOR MODIFICATIONS.** Chefs can get heavy-handed with prep ("hmm, this could use more butter—where's my shovel?"), so don't hesitate to ask for sauces and dressings on the side. In addition, request "easy on the oil" and "no butter." Always ask politely, of course—like any professional, chefs take pride in what they do. But in the end it's your health you're protecting, so get your food the way you need it.

4. **STICK TO FLIPPING.** Even if you modify a restaurant dish, it will likely have more calories than a home-prepared meal. Expect that when ordering. Stick to flipping as much as you can, don't order multiple courses (restaurant appetizers can be as caloric as a normal meal), and don't feel compelled to clean your plate.

shop yourself skinny

WITH RACHEL'S MVPS (MOST VALUED PRODUCTS)

your zero-guesswork, aisle-by-aisle visual shop guide

Just grab and go!

Yes, I'm a shopping addict. I'm not talking clothes or accessories—okay, maybe accessories. I'm talking food, of course! Whenever I'm in a new city, I can't resist popping into the local stores to see what's on their shelves. My scouting trips help me to understand why so many of my patients get confused when it comes to buying food. In every single store I immediately see two big issues:

1. There are more choices than ever. Our parents grew up with a few brands that became household names. Today new food products from companies we've never heard of get introduced every day.

2. There's more misinformation than ever. It seems as if every package makes health or sustainability claims. Only the hardest of the hard-core junk foods don't make any claims, so they actually seem the most honest!

In other words, it's not the shopping, it's the guesswork that kills us.

I could write a long shopping list for you—but you know the saying, a picture is worth a thousand words? It's true! So in the next few pages, you'll find *visual shopping guides* of my superstar Most Valuable Products (MVPs)—items that should be in everyone's fridge, pantry, and fruit bowl. At one glance you'll know exactly what to buy—no more guesswork. Zip. Zero. *Nada.* I've done all the label-reading legwork, so you know you're picking the right foods to get to your weight and health goals. It's like having your own personal dietitian take you shopping!

Of course, there are many more MVPs than what are pictured here. Consider this your must-have starter kit. For the latest updates, check out my Facebook page (www.facebook.com/RachelBeller).

And by the way, I do get samples from the food companies, but not a single dime. My recommendations are based 100 percent on my unbiased analysis—in fact, I wind up rejecting far more than I ever select.

P.S. If you can't find these exact products, don't fret! You can always go online and find everything (even cheaper), or just look for the closest thing to it and follow my guidelines from Part 1. And of course, organic is always preferred when possible.

Enough words: Are you ready to get visual? Then grab your wallet, your keys, and your must-wear accessories, and let's go shopping!

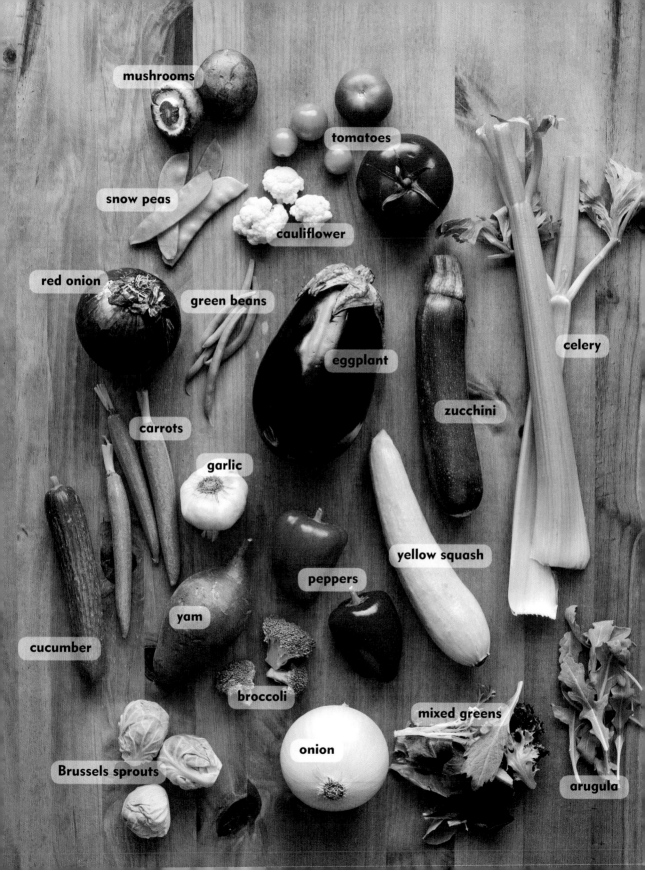

mushrooms

tomatoes

snow peas

cauliflower

celery

red onion

green beans

eggplant

zucchini

carrots

garlic

yellow squash

peppers

yam

cucumber

broccoli

mixed greens

onion

Brussels sprouts

arugula

what to grab
from the produce aisle

I like to tell my patients to think of the empty shopping cart as their empty stomach. Keeping with the Flip-It philosophy, they should fill it with the "good stuff" first, and by that I mean antioxidant- and fiber-rich fruits (my favorite candy!) and vegetables.

To help you get started, I focused this shopping list on basics that are available year-round and are used in many of my suggested meals and snacks. And, of course, you can add anything else you like.

So here's my weekly veg and fruit hit list. I always have these on hand to take the guess-work out of making meals—and to take the guesswork out of shopping in the first place.

Vegetables

- Bagged prewashed mixed greens or baby spinach
- Arugula
- Carrots
- Broccoli
- Cauliflower
- Zucchini

- Yellow squash
- Onions (red and yellow)
- Eggplant
- Tomatoes
- Cucumbers
- Celery

- Garlic
- Bell peppers
- Brussels sprouts
- Yams
- Mushrooms (any)
- Snow peas
- Green beans

VEG EXTRA CREDIT!

Want to upgrade the nutritional value of your foods—and add some flavor in the process? (Who would say no to that?) Then add any of my 14 favorite nutritional boosters to your meals. Don't feel compelled to buy all of these every week—just use them frequently.

- **BROCCOLI SPROUTS** This all-star booster provides 20 to 50 times the amount of sulforaphane, a phytochemical that can reduce risk of developing cancer, as broccoli florets. Just 1 ounce (about 1 tablespoon) of sprouts contains as much cancer-fighting sulforaphane as 1½ pounds of broccoli.

- **RED CABBAGE** Want to make your salads super? For about $1.50 you can buy a bag of shredded red cabbage filled with incredible cancer-fighting properties (indole-3-carbinol).

- **SAUERKRAUT** Yogurt has some competition in the probiotics world! Betcha didn't know that sauerkraut is a dairy-free source of stomach-friendly, immunity-boosting probiotics, as well as vitamins and minerals. The fermentation of the cabbage provides these nutritional benefits. The key to getting the most live and active cultures is to buy the naturally fermented refrigerated varieties, as heat can kill off some of the live and active cultures. Tip: Before eating, rinse under cold water to cut the sodium.

- **NORI (DRIED SEAWEED SHEETS)** Widely available (even Walmart carries them!), and for just 15 to 20 cents per sheet, nori isn't just a sushi wrapper, it's a nutritional steal. Seaweed's wealth of minerals will enhance your hair and skin, so be sure to keep a pack within sight. (Check out my easy Salmon Hand Rolls on page 117.)

- **WATERCRESS** Watercress offers loads of protective benefits—including reduced cancer risk—at just 4 calories a cup. Studies reveal that watercress may reduce breast cancer risk, along with many other nutritional claims to fame.

- **BASIL** Not only do basil leaves enhance soups, salads, and more, they also pack both antibacterial and antioxidant properties—with some evidence also linking basil consumption to cancer prevention.

- **OREGANO** Italian food wouldn't be Italian food without oregano. Even better, oregano is another significant source of "antis," with forty-two times more antioxidant power than apples and four times more than blueberries.

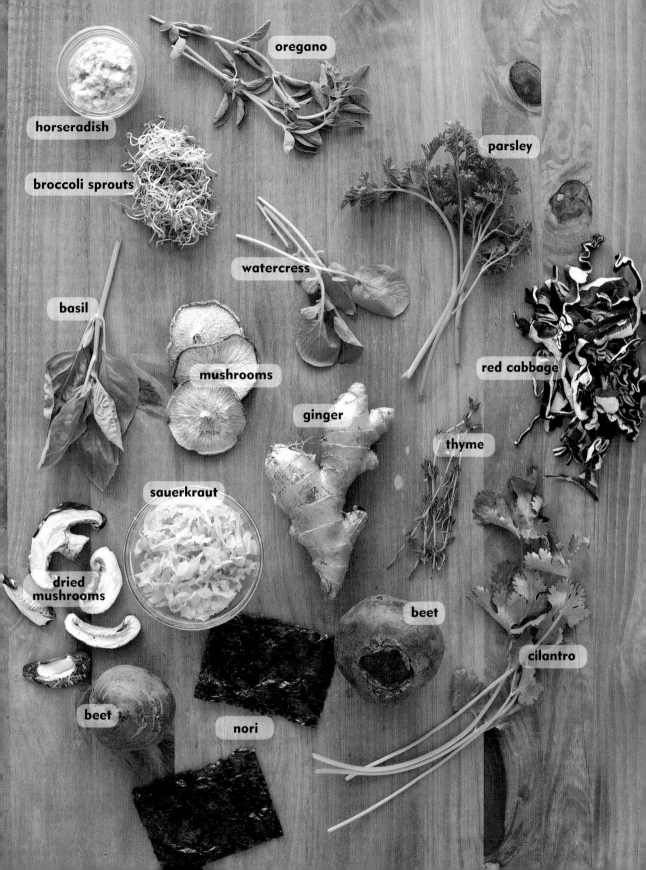

horseradish

oregano

parsley

broccoli sprouts

watercress

basil

mushrooms

red cabbage

ginger

thyme

sauerkraut

dried mushrooms

beet

cilantro

beet

nori

- **THYME** Yes, thyme is on your side. Sorry, cheap joke, I know, but it's true: Thyme is a powerful antiseptic, antibacterial, and strong antioxidant.

- **PARSLEY** I like to think of parsley as a "multivitamin" loaded with antioxidants. It's also a handy diuretic. Parsley de-bloats and flushes excess water out of the body, which is a plus when you're trying to squeeze into your favorite jeans.

- **CILANTRO** This tasty source of iron and magnesium can help fight anemia. It can also relieve stomach gas as an overall digestive aid, and it may even lower cholesterol.

- **GINGER** Hot and exotic ginger has it all: It works as an anti-inflammatory, fights nausea, aids digestion, and is a potential fat burner.

- **DEHYDRATED MUSHROOMS** You gotta love mushrooms, and not just their meaty flavor. Mushrooms in general pack protein, probiotics, antioxidants, and anti-inflammatory properties. But the drying process improves overall nutritional value.

- **BEETS** For thousands of years, people have used beets as a folk remedy. Just a little bit adds a sweet and nutritious punch to your salad. In addition to fresh, look for presteamed beets in your local produce section or no-sugar-added varieties in jars.

- **HORSERADISH** With horseradish, a little bit goes a long way—and I'm not just talking about the mega-potent kick that clears your sinuses! Horseradish contains intensely concentrated amounts of glucosinolates, a compound that forms phytochemicals that can lower your risk of cancer. In fact, horseradish contains more glucosinolates than most cruciferous vegetables, so just a dash will do the trick. (That said, eat as much as you can handle.) Tip: Mix horseradish with Greek yogurt and lime juice to tame the kick and create a yummy dressing for chicken and veggies. In the supermarket you'll find fresh horseradish in little jars near the refrigerated pickles.

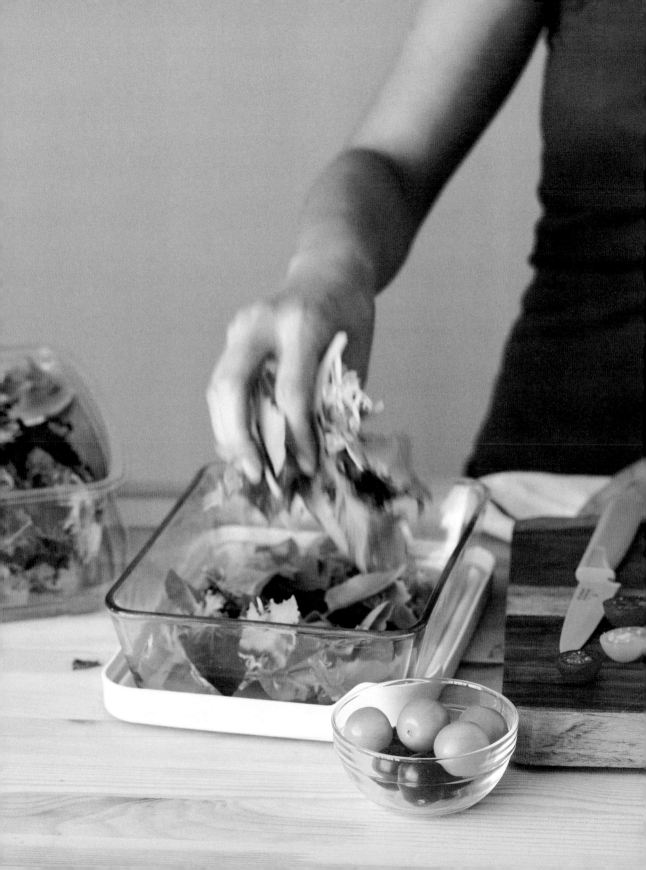

FRESH HERBS—LOVE 'EM!

Herbs add so much flavor to dishes without resorting to calorie-heavy sauces or oils (another reason I included herbs in my list of "meal boosters"). But a lot of people just don't know what the heck to do with them. So here are some ideas:

- Basil + sautéed shallots + grape tomatoes =
  an amazing topping for fish or chicken or even stirred into quinoa

- Dill + lemon + minced garlic + dollop of Greek yogurt =
  a delicious dip for crudités or sauce for grilled salmon

- Cilantro + lime zest and juice + chopped scallions =
  a fab topping for fish tacos (also great stirred into a bit of brown rice)

Experiment!

Fruit

Again, any kind of fruit is a go in my book! But these staples are available year-round—and the ones I always pick up at the market. Stock up your fruit bowl.

- Pears
- Apples (red and green)
- Oranges
- Tangerines
- Blueberries
- Strawberries
- Blackberries
- Raspberries
- Bananas
- Red grapes

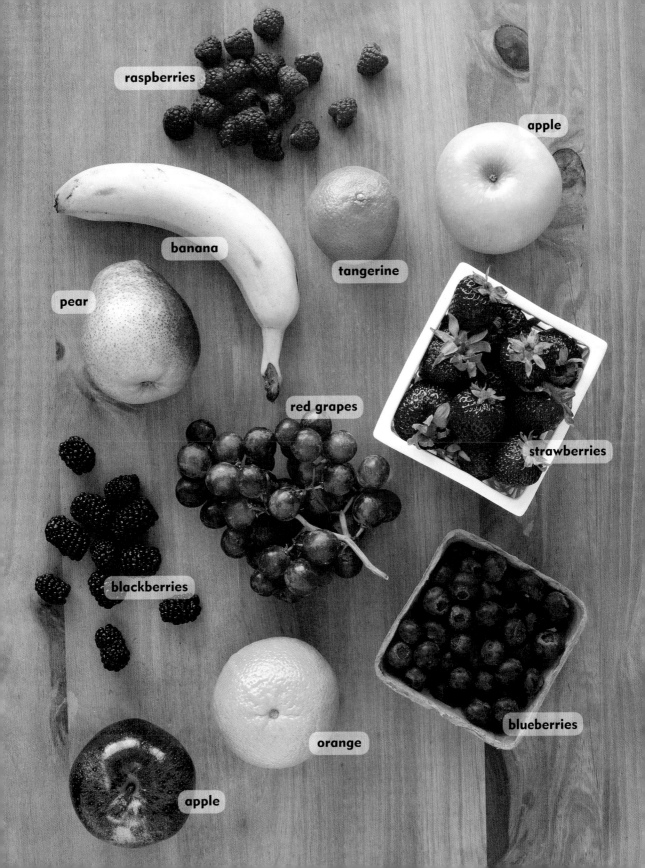

raspberries

apple

banana

tangerine

pear

red grapes

strawberries

blackberries

blueberries

orange

apple

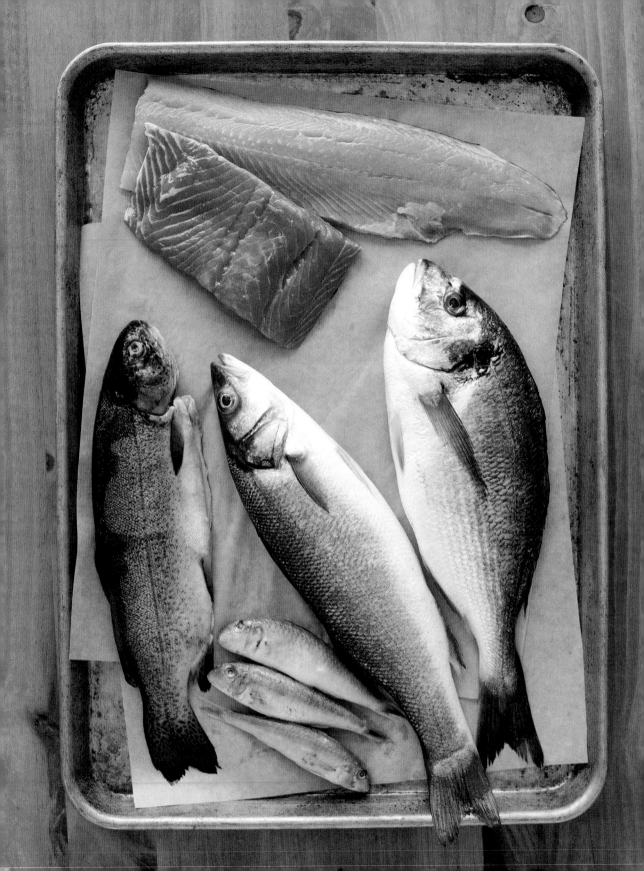

your best fish
and seafood bets

Whoever first said that there are always more fish in the sea was probably staring at a super-market fish counter. I bet you've had the same feeling. You hear you should eat more fish, but you encounter all these requirements and choices: avoid mercury, get more omega-3s, farmed or wild, and does it come from sustainable sources? How does anyone make a smart decision?

So you head over to the canned section and you see entire schools of tuna. Suddenly you feel like you need a school of your own just to learn how to shop.

That's why I put together this brief handy section on fish and other seafood.

Canned Fish

Can't figure out your counterattack? Don't sweat it. Canned fish is less expensive and some-times can be more healthful than the fresh catches. Many fish (like wild salmon) are seasonal, so more get caught than can be sold at once. The rest gets canned or frozen, giving you an incredible price point.

So stock up on canned fish! Here's what you should get.

- LOW-MERCURY ALBACORE TUNA (can or pouch): Wild Planet, Raincoast, and Ameri-can Tuna are my go-to brands for canned albacore. Their tuna is sustainably caught and contains approximately *six times* the omega-3s as conventional tuna brands. Plus, these specific brands are low in mercury because the fish are smaller in size. Although they cost an extra dollar or so per can, you get so much more bang for your buck! These cans give you a full 5 ounces of tuna in each can, whereas conventional brands add water or vegetable oil so you're getting only 3.5 ounces of tuna and 1.5 ounces of additive. Also, you can go online and get these brands way cheaper, or look for Wild Planet at your local grocery and warehouse stores. Yes, going wild is becoming mainstream and is within reach.

- SUSTAINABLE SEAS TUNA: This is not as high in omega-3s as the low-mercury albacore brands, but it's still sustainably caught and higher in omega-3s and lower in mercury than conventional brands yet costs practically the same.

- WILD SALMON (can or pouch): My ultimate cheap and easy omega-3 fish solution. Any variety will do, but best bet is to look for sockeye salmon on the label, as it's the *crème de la crème* of salmon in terms of omega-3 fats. Any market has it.

- SARDINES: If you're even considering sardines, I'm taking that as an open door and sticking my foot in, because sardines are one of the best foods for you: naturally low in mercury, high in omega-3s, vitamin D, calcium, B_{12}, and coenzyme Q_{10}. You can

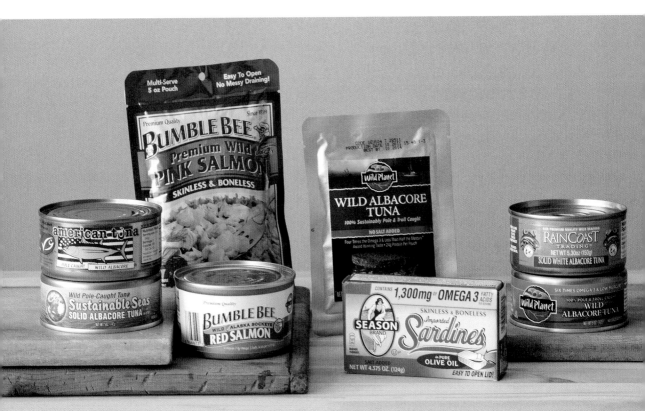

eat the whole tin for only 150 to 200 calories. Plus, they're superaffordable! Stick to canned in water or olive oil. Tip: Canned sardines pair well with flatbread and a smear of Dijon mustard.

CHEW ON THIS FOR EXTRA CREDIT: Although wild salmon and sardines usually come boneless, I recommend trying the bone-in kind. The bones are soft and edible, and will give your body the best calcium boost it can ask for.

SEAFOOD MERCURY AND OMEGA-3 CONTENT

Low mercury/ High omega-3 A total go!	Moderate mercury Go easy.	High mercury Try to avoid.
Wild salmon (fresh and canned)	Sea bass (black)	Shark
Trout	Halibut	Swordfish
Crab	Mahi mahi	King mackerel
Black cod (Alaska/Canada)	Lobster	Tilefish (golden bass or golden snapper)
Flounder	Canned chunk light tuna	Grouper
Pacific sole		Sea bass (Chilean)
Shrimp		Orange roughy
Canned low-mercury tuna brands		Tuna (ahi)
Sardines		Canned white albacore tuna
Scallops (low-mercury but moderate in omega-3)		

From the Natural Resources Defense Council (www.nrdc.org/health/effects/mercury/guide.asp)

what to look for when buying meat and poultry

I designed my Protein GPS to help you navigate your way through the maze of protein options. Now let's get even more focused: What should you do in the meat section of the supermarket? After all, that's where everything looks the same—and you'll find little to no helpful info on the packaging.

If you're like many of my patients, you've put your meat shopping on autopilot: You buzz over to the same section of the meat case, scan the Little Three (chicken, turkey, and beef), and grab the same things every time. Now it's time to change direction.

Pay attention here: My recommendations may differ from what you're used to, but I guarantee that you'll bring home leaner, healthier choices of the Little Three—plus pork.

SKINLESS CHICKEN BREAST Go USDA-certified organic! That means the chickens were raised "free range" on organic feed and not exposed to fertilizers, pesticides, antibiotics, or other potentially harmful chemicals. (The same isn't true of poultry simply labeled "free range.")

SKINLESS TURKEY BREAST Same rule applies here as with chicken.

LEAN GROUND TURKEY Supermarkets label poultry and other meat by their "percent lean." That can be misleading. For example, ground turkey that's "85 percent lean" sounds good, but if you stop to think about it, that means it's 15 percent fat! For a 4-ounce portion,

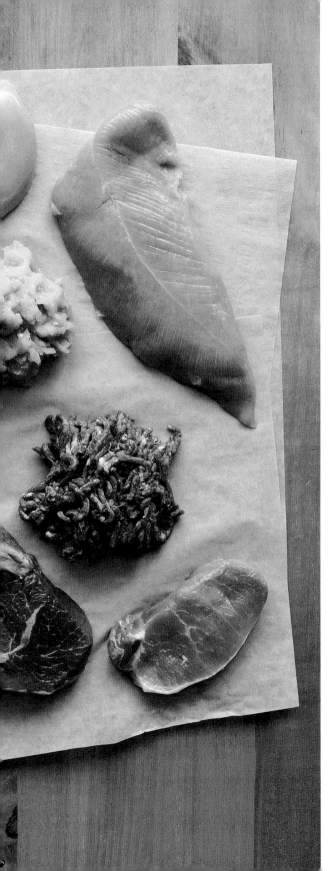

you're looking at around 17 grams of fat, 5 of it saturated. So go for turkey that's at least 93 percent lean.

NITRATE-FREE TURKEY COLD CUTS Any brand will do, as long as the label specifies *nitrate-free*—meaning the meat is cured without this potentially carcinogenic chemical.

GROUND 95-PERCENT LEAN GRASS-FED BEEF The cow's diet—grass-only, versus one that includes corn and other grains—affects the nutrients and fats in the meat itself. Grass-fed beef also tends to have less fat and more omega-3s and antioxidants than traditional beef. Yes, it's pricier, but you'll likely be eating so much less red meat than before—and more proteins like eggs and beans, which are super-inexpensive—that it will more than even out!

"ROUND" CUTS OF BEEF If you spot this word—as in eye round, top round, or bottom round—you're looking at a lean cut of red meat.

"LOIN" CUTS OF BEEF As with "round" cuts, those with "loin" in the name—such as sirloin and tenderloin—are also lean.

"LOIN" CUTS OF PORK Tenderloin and loin chops are also your best bets when it comes to pork. In fact, a serving of tenderloin has fewer calories and even slightly less fat than the same portion of chicken breast.

next stop, aisle b: beans!

Preparing most beans from scratch can take hours and hours—just not realistic for most people I know (including myself). So I've included only the easiest bean options here. They're good-to-go and huge on nutrition. This is fast food at its best!

BLACK BELUGA LENTILS All lentils are great (brown, French green, yellow, red), but my new favorite is black beluga. The black color comes from anthocyanin pigment, which also functions as an incredible antioxidant. Black beluga lentils are especially delicious and petite, and they maintain their round shape, which makes them perfect for salads. Plus, most health food stores carry them. They take about twenty minutes to cook—less time than it takes to find parking at the mall.

MUNG BEANS Also twenty minutes to cook. If you aren't familiar with mung beans, they're worth getting to know! They are a nutritional powerhouse and widely available in most markets. The key is not to overcook them, as that will reduce their nutritional value and make them mushy.

SPROUTED MUNG BEANS OR LENTILS (DRIED) Being "sprouted" means they take just five minutes to cook and are easy to digest. What's not to like?

EDAMAME You'll find these in the freezer section of the market (both in the pod and shelled). I always keep some organic edamame in the freezer for a quick protein fix.

CANNED EDEN AND AMY'S BEANS (MULTIPLE VARIETIES) These great brands use BPA-free cans. Rinse the beans well to reduce the sodium and gas-inducing compounds.

MEXICAN TAKEOUT All the work—from degassing to cooking—has been done for you, and for not much more than the price of the same amount of canned beans.

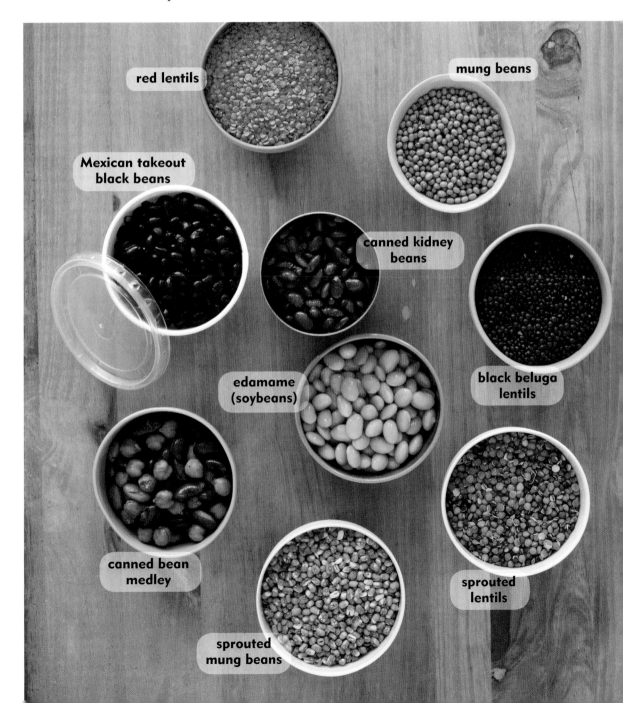

eggs, tofu, and other refrigerated proteins

Eggs

Eggs are an incredible deal: protein, choline, and omega-3s—in one inexpensive, low-calorie package. But I do have some important shopping pointers for you.

OMEGA-3–RICH EGGS Lately the attention has been turned up on "omega-3–enhanced" or "enriched" eggs. And here's where you gotta watch the labels—and your wallet. *All* eggs contain omega-3s—approximately 50 milligrams each. So if the front of the package boasts "50 milligrams of omega-3s," it's saying, "These are regular eggs." Truly enhanced or enriched eggs come from chickens fed omega-3–rich foods like flax oil, flaxseed, walnuts, fish meal, or algae. Those eggs will have around 100 milligrams of omega-3s each. Look for enriched eggs that contain DHA, the omega-3 essential fatty acid normally found in fish, which is worth paying a little extra for.

EGG WHITES (CARTON) In contrast to fresh egg whites, eggs in the carton have been heated to pasteurize them, which takes some of the fluffy *oomph* out of them and makes them less desirable for recipes that require rising. But egg whites in the carton are a great fast-food item to keep in your fridge if you don't like to separate your own egg whites (I do!). You can cut some of the fat and calories in omelets and scrambled eggs by using one whole egg and three or four whites. You get the choline from the whole egg but still keep the calories low thanks to the whites.

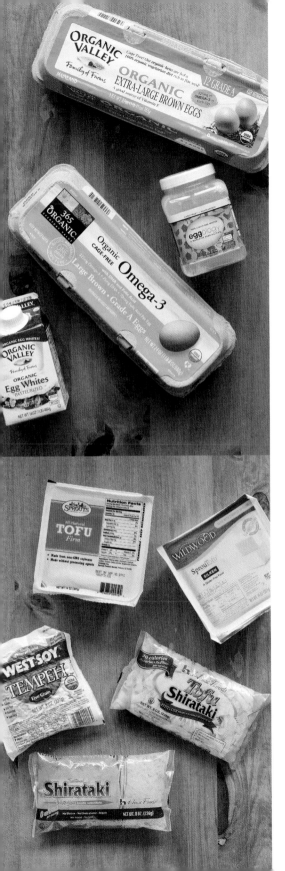

Tofu

Whatever shape or flavor of tofu you like, follow this one critical rule: Go organic! Soybeans offer a lot of health benefits, but they're often genetically modified and grown with a lot of pesticides. By spending a few cents more, you can go organic and GMO-free—well-worth the expense! My recs:

SPROUTED ORGANIC TOFU Not only does it contain more nutrients than regular organic tofu but because it's made from sprouted beans, it's easier to digest. (Not that regular tofu is necessarily hard on the stomach, but sensitive tummies might appreciate the sprouted variety.)

ORGANIC TEMPEH Add tempeh to a variety of recipes, including soups and tomato sauce. Or you can simply season it and eat it crumbled or as a burger patty. Because tempeh is made from fermented whole soybeans, it's easy to digest. It also contains more protein and fiber than tofu, but it does have more calories, so you gotta watch portions. You can find organic tempeh in the refrigerated section of most health food stores.

SHIRATAKI NOODLES Found at most markets for less than $1.50 a bag, these soybean-based noodles are super-low in calories and carbs (half a bag has 20 calories, 3 grams of carbs, and 2 grams of fiber!), and the konjac fiber (a fiber derived from the konjac plant) found in them may lower cholesterol and help keep your blood sugar in check. Cooking tip: Make your pasta with a 50/50 split of whole wheat pasta and shirataki noodles, or add the shirataki noodles to stir-fry dishes.

cereals, breads, pastas, grains, and snacks

Cereals

Picking a cereal when we were kids was so easy: You just found the box with the best toy in it and hope Mom didn't object. But after two bites, all that sugar would make your head spin!

Today cereals make our heads spin from all the choices on the shelves—and all that hype and fine print on the boxes. So let's take out the spinning and turn to winning: Here are my faves from the Great Wall of Cereal in the supermarket.

Base Cereals

Base cereals are the must-haves in your cereal bowl, as they meet all of my criteria for cereal (see page 24). Enjoy them all on their own—or, if you need more fun in your bowl, use them with my suggested mixer cereals. But be sure to have at least ½ cup of one of these base cereals to get your fiber insurance.

KELLOGG'S ALL-BRAN OR BENEFIT NUTRITION SIMPLY FIBER CINNAMON These high-fiber cereals are for the purist at heart. They contain very few ingredients and lots of fiber. Adding cinnamon and berries kicks the flavor up a notch.

NATURE'S PATH ORGANIC SMART BRAN Tastes way better than it looks! Smart Bran is not only organic; it's also rich in soluble fiber from psyllium husk and oat bran. Although it's a great

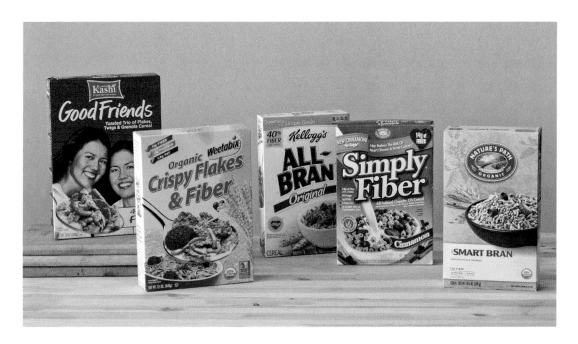

base for cereal mixing, it's also a great stand-alone cereal. The only drawback: It's hard to find outside of health food stores (easier and cheaper online).

KASHI GOOD FRIENDS HIGH FIBER CEREAL The sugar in the cereal is at the absolute max of what I recommend—but it's a great-tasting high fiber cereal that can be found in most supermarkets.

WEETABIX ORGANIC CRISPY FLAKES & FIBER Everyone loves the taste of this Weetabix variety. The serving size is a bit larger than a cup, but the calories are still in check. It tastes amazing, offers up 11 grams of fiber, and is relatively inexpensive. The downside: It's mainly available online (Amazon). The upside: You'll end up paying less than you would at the market.

Mixer Cereals

If some of the base cereals are too "saw dust-y" for you, try a little creative mixology. (No, I'm not talking martinis for breakfast.) Just remember this easy fiber-fun equation: base cereal + mixer cereal = fiber with a twist of playfulness! Be creative—mix and match different cereals to fill your bowl with flavor, style, and texture. A friendly reminder: Your mix should have at least 10 grams of fiber and no more than 10 grams of sugar or 200 calories per cup. Here are a few of my favorite mixer cereals.

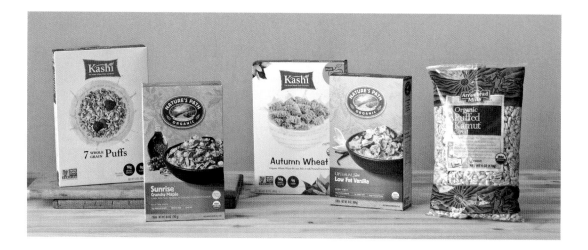

NATURE'S PATH MAPLE SUNRISE OR NATURE'S PATH OPTIMUM SLIM VANILLA These mixer cereals are winners with absolutely everyone. High-fiber base cereals work well undercover when mixed with one of these, since they give you a few different textures in one box—and are totally tasty.

KASHI AUTUMN WHEAT Totally kid-approved, and how could I not fall in love with its ultra-short ingredient list (just three!)? Since the 1 cup serving doesn't dish up 10 grams of fiber, use this as a mixer with a base cereal, or simply add a fiber boost (fruit or chia seeds) to fill the fiber gap.

HUNTING AND GATHERING TIPS

If you can't find these items in your local market, or at a price you like, don't throw in the towel!

First go online: Amazon, for example, offers a wealth of exotic and healthy foods, often at store-beating prices.

Still no luck? Still no worries! My recommendations also serve as guides; try to find something similar. (Be sure to read the labels carefully.)

My goal is for you to achieve a better *you*. That means your personal winning formula might vary a little, but close enough is usually good enough!

KAMUT PUFFS (ANY BRAND, LIKE ARROWHEAD MILLS) OR KASHI 7 WHOLE GRAIN PUFFS These are for people who like volume in their bowls, so I've dubbed them "volumizers." At only 50 to 70 calories per cup, both cereals are also great as a snack (see page 76).

Oatmeal

My personal a.m. favorite is to go with the real deal: steel-cut oats! The grains are whole and chewy, and therefore they digest slower than rolled oats, and most certainly slower than instant oatmeal packs. So get picky about your oatmeal. And remember that with most of these options, you'll need to add a fiber boost (see page 27) to get your a.m. fiber fix. Here are my top oatmeal recommendations.

MCCANN'S STEEL-CUT OATMEAL (OR ANY BRAND) It takes a while to cook—30 to 40 minutes—but it's worth the wait. Time-saving tip: At night, boil the oatmeal in water for 1 minute, then turn off the heat and cover the pot. In the morning, turn the heat back on and cook for an additional 5 to 7 minutes . . . done! Make extra and refrigerate or freeze it for those weekday morning rushes.

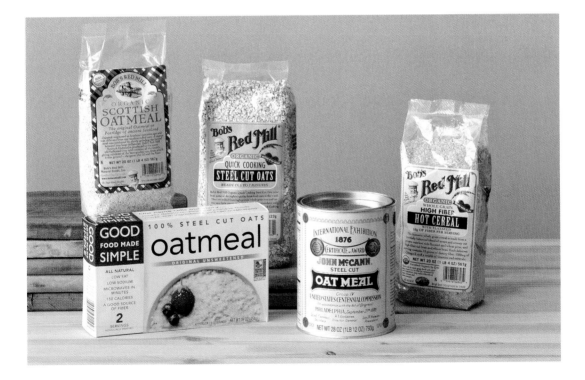

BOB'S RED MILL QUICK COOKING STEEL CUT OATS Same as the slower cooked steel cut oats but the oats have been made into smaller pieces, which allows for shorter cook time. Just 5 to 7 minutes and you're ready to eat!

BOB'S RED MILL HIGH FIBER HOT CEREAL What I love about this hot cereal is that it delivers 10 grams of fiber per serving. If you like a hot cereal with a fiber boost but chia is not your thing, then this is your ticket. Add a diced apple or a cup of berries and you're looking at 14 grams of fiber. This cereal is a blend of stone-ground oats, flax, wheat germ, oat bran, and wheat bran.

GOOD FOOD MADE SIMPLE 100% STEEL-CUT FROZEN OATMEAL Ideal when you literally need to get breakfast on the table in two minutes—it comes in precooked, preportioned pouches that you just heat and enjoy. If you can't find this particular brand in your freezer section, look for a similar unsweetened or low-sugar frozen variety. I sometimes enjoy this as my 150 calorie p.m. snack at work.

SCOTTISH OATMEAL Oatmeal isn't just for breakfast anymore. This variety is stone ground, which makes for a creamy hot cereal that's soothing and comforting. Try eating ½ cup an hour or two before bedtime (see page 83).

The Big, Bad Bread Aisle—and a Selection of Whole Grains

Want to find the real nutritious deal in the ever-baffling bread section? You'll have to read all the labels and give every loaf my Squeeze Test (see page 30) . . . or you can simply buy from my list here.

MESTEMACHER NATURAL WHOLE RYE You can usually spot this bread on the bottom shelf because it's dense and doesn't look like your typical loaf of bread. Beyond touch, this is truly a whole grain bread—you can actually *see* the whole rye kernels. Each slice contains 120 to 130 calories—almost as much as 2 average bread slices—so break it in half. Tip: Be sure to toast it. Pairs best with a cheese spread and sliced tomatoes.

FOOD FOR LIFE EZEKIEL BREADS Great hearty taste and my go-to faves. It's organic, flourless, and sprouting gives you more vitamins and allows for better absorption of nutrients. This looks like something you'd only find at health food stores, but nowadays you can find it almost anywhere. The cinnamon raisin is a total treat: Toast it and it tastes like dessert! Tip: Best kept refrigerated.

MILTON'S WHOLE GRAIN PLUS Call this one "middle of the road" bread. Not too firm, yet passes my Squeeze Test. There are visible grains and flaxseed within the slices, and the best part is that it's totally kid-approved. It has one manufactured fiber, but it's less than 2 percent of the ingredients list. Each slice has 80 calories and 4 grams of fiber.

RUDI'S 7 GRAIN WITH FLAX If you're at a health food store and you spot this bread—*grab it*! It's got all kinds of grains within each slice and there is no need to toast it. If you're craving a half tuna sandwich as your afternoon snack, this one will make the grade and then some. Delish!

OROWEAT/ARNOLD/BROWNBERRY WHOLE GRAIN HEALTHY MULTI-GRAIN If you can't find any of the other suggested breads, you can buy this at any market. I've dubbed it an "introductory bread" for those trying to work up from white to whole grain since its texture isn't super firm and grainy. The upside: It doesn't easily roll into a marble, and you can still spot little pieces of grains within.

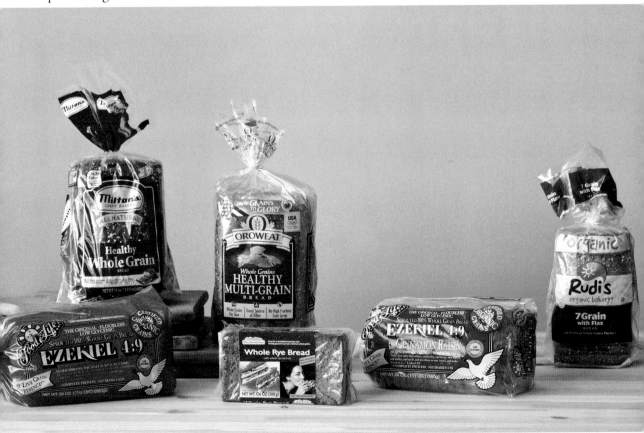

BREAD LABELS DECODED!

Remember when bread was so simple our grandparents called it a "staple"? Now we need staples just to keep the pages of ingredients together!

Even worse, today you need a translator to tell you what half those ingredients mean—and what they'll do to you.

That's why I created this quick guide to bread labels, especially if you can't find one of my recommended brands.

The "Good" Bread—That Isn't

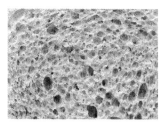

Not a visible piece of grain in sight! Easily rolls into a marble—Squeeze Test fail!

And don't be fooled by grain claims on the package. It could be 7 grain, 10 grain, or *200 grain*—but the fact is you only need one and it should be a "whole" grain! Let's take a look at the ingredients.

Ingredients: WHOLE WHEAT FLOUR, UNBLEACHED ENRICHED WHEAT FLOUR [FLOUR, MALTED BARLEY FLOUR, REDUCED IRON, NIACIN, THIAMIN MONONITRATE (VITAMIN B1), RIBOFLAVIN (VITAMIN B2), FOLIC ACID, WATER, WHEAT GLUTEN, WHEAT FIBER, YEAST, SUGAR, CELLULOSE FIBER, INULIN (CHICKORY ROOT FIBER), POLYDEXTROSE, SUNFLOWER SEEDS, WHEAT, RYE, MOLASSES, WHEAT PROTEIN ISOLATE, SALT, GROUND CORN, CULTURED DEXTROSE AND MALTODEXTRIN (A NATURAL PRESERVATIVE), RAISIN JUICE CONCENTRATE, BUCKWHEAT, DATEM, MONOGLYCERIDES, BROWN RICE, OATS, TRITICALE, CITRIC ACID, BARLEY, FLAXSEED, MILLET, CALCIUM SULFATE, GRAIN VINEGAR, STEVIA EXTRACT (A NATURAL SWEETENER), SOY LECITHIN, CALCIUM CARBONATE, NUTS [WALNUTS AND/OR HAZELNUTS (FILBERTS) AND/OR ALMONDS], RICE PROTEIN, WHEY, SOY FLOUR, NONFAT MILK.

Sure, the numbers fit your requirements: 80 calories and 4 grams of fiber. But wait . . . don't forget that ingredient list! Whole wheat flour *is* the first ingredient on the list—but the second one is a *refined white flour* (unbleached enriched wheat flour). It also contains not one, but *five* types of manufactured fiber (cellulose fiber, inulin, polydextrose, wheat fiber, and maltodextrin).

And while there's nothing wrong with molasses, its only purpose here is to color the bread so it *looks* healthier.

The "Better" Bread

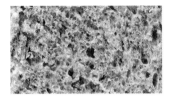

I see some visible pieces of grain, and it resists serious squishing—a good sign. But let's decode the ingredients.

Ingredients: WHOLE WHEAT FLOUR, WATER, WHEAT GLUTEN, BROWN RICE, CORNMEAL, OATS, CRACKED WHEAT, WHEAT BRAN, YEAST, CELLULOSE FIBER, SOYBEAN OIL, GOLDEN FLAX, BLACK & WHITE SESAME SEEDS, QUINOA FLOUR, SALT, DATEM, CALCIUM SULFATE, POPPY SEEDS, GRAIN VINEGAR, SOY LECITHIN, CITRIC ACID, CALCIUM CARBONATE, NUTS [WALNUTS AND/OR HAZELNUTS (FILBERTS) AND/OR ALMONDS], WHEY.

Although whole wheat flour is the first ingredient (more nutrient rich than refined white flour), it's still less than ideal. But we are looking better since it has pieces of grains within the slices, and only one manufactured fiber. If your options are limited, this is fine.

The "Best in Show" Bread

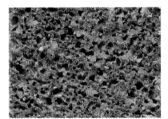

It passes my Squeeze Test with flying colors, the fiber and calories are a go, and there are big visible grains within the slice, not just coating the outside. Let's just double-check the ingredients.

Ingredients: ORGANIC SPROUTED WHOLE WHEAT, FILTERED WATER, ORGANIC MALTED BARLEY, ORGANIC SPROUTED WHOLE MILLET, ORGANIC SPROUTED WHOLE BARLEY, ORGANIC SPROUTED WHOLE LENTILS, ORGANIC SPROUTED WHOLE SOYBEANS, ORGANIC SPROUTED WHOLE SPELT, FRESH YEAST, ORGANIC WHEAT GLUTEN, SEA SALT.

Chock-full of goodness—and make that *organic* goodness. The o-word comes up eight times and the w-word (whole) comes up six times! It's completely flourless for better blood sugar regulation.

Notice: No ingredients you'd need a chemist to pronounce. All completely identifiable stuff here and no faux fibers. When it comes to bread, this is one of your best bets!

Tortillas and Pitas

Tortillas and pitas are so tasty and versatile. You can use them to wrap just about anything, not only the traditional bean/cheese/meat combos. For example, grilled veg taste great in a tortilla with a touch of goat cheese. Or a pita can be stuffed with fresh cucumbers and hummus.

FOOD FOR LIFE EZEKIEL SPROUTED GRAIN TORTILLAS AND CORN TORTILLAS I consider the sprouted varieties as the top tier of tortillas. They're organic and chewy, and everything is "whole."

They come in small and large sizes, but just know that the large size counts as nearly two bread-slice equivalents. As an alternative to the sprouted grain, go for the corn.

LOW-CARB TORTILLAS AND PITAS If the whole grain varieties don't excite you and you really want that voluminous chewy carb texture, you can choose from a number of low-carb options. Note: The primary fiber source for most of these products will be manufactured fibers, so don't bank on these for your daily fiber goal.

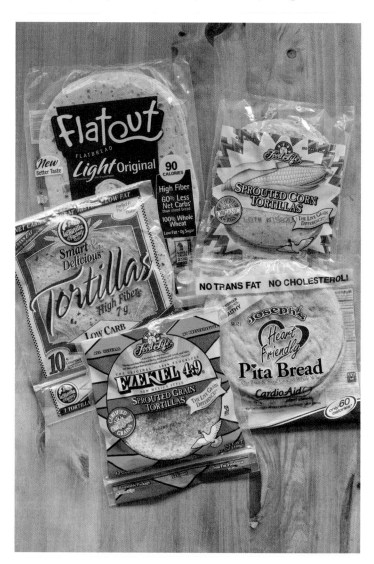

Other Whole Grains and Whole Grain Products

You know the expression "amber waves of grain"? That's what you'll find when you hit the supermarket these days. And not just the usual wheat and rice either. You'll discover all sorts of varieties that you might have never heard of. But don't stress about it: The beauty of grains is that they all offer protein, fiber, vitamins, and minerals and are super-easy on your wallet. I love 'em all. Here are a few you should definitely check out.

1. FARRO Very similar in texture to barley, this grain makes a great side dish. Cooking is a cinch: Just boil for 20 to 30 minutes until tender. It's a protein superstar that contains fewer calories and more fiber than the same amount of quinoa. Tip: Buy semi-pearled instead of pearled, as it still has the bran intact.

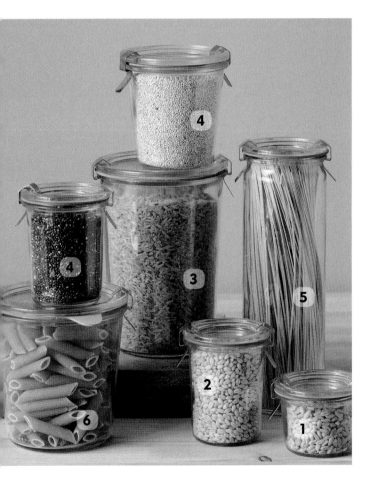

2. WHEAT BERRIES These are wheat kernels with only the hull removed. You can serve them as a side dish or add them to stews for more texture and nutrients. Note: Soft wheat berries are lower in protein and gluten than the hard variety.

3. BROWN RICE Forget white rice, which has been processed and refined to death, losing nutrients. Go with the original brown. If you prefer fluffy rice, use long grain; if you prefer stickier rice, go short grain. Tip: Soaking brown rice (30 minutes to overnight) before cooking increases absorption and digestibility of the nutrients.

4. QUINOA (REGULAR AND RED) Quinoa is booming in popularity because it's a complete protein, it's gluten-free, and it doesn't take long to cook. It's also extremely versatile. Use it as a side dish, an oatmeal substitute, or as a protein enhancement for salads. Tip: Rinse it before cooking in order to remove the bitter saponin coating.

5. SOBA These thin Japanese noodles are made from buckwheat, which contains antioxidants, magnesium, B vitamins, and choline. Add some stir-fry veg for extra fiber, or use them in cold dishes like salads. Seek out 100 percent buckwheat versions.

6. WHOLE WHEAT PASTA Start replacing the regular white bleached (semolina) pasta in your diet with whole wheat. You'll get more protein and fiber (about 7 grams protein and 2 to 4 grams fiber per 1 cup cooked). For maximum benefits, cook it al dente—keeps your blood sugar steadier (see page 230).

Crackers

When you crave that satisfying *crunch,* forget evil potato chips. Go crackers—especially if you need an emergency at-your-desk breakfast or snack (just add a sliced apple and some string cheese). Here are my favorites. I generally stick with large flatbreads, not the smaller squares, because tasty bite-size crackers make it too easy to lose control!

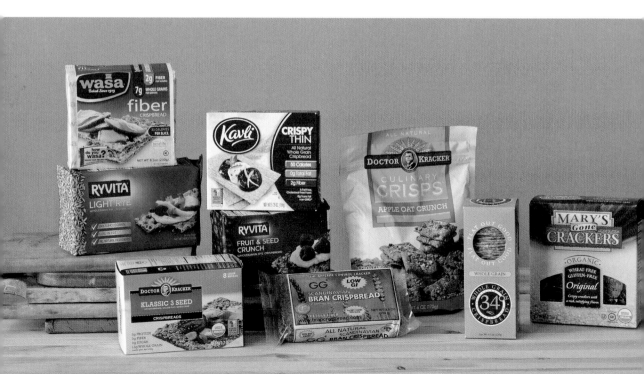

FIBER CRISPBREADS—WASA, KAVLI, AND RYVITA These are the Cadillacs of crackers. That's because the ingredient lists for each celebrate the less-is-more mentality—delivering simple, pure, crunchy whole grain goodness. Any variety will do!

RYVITA FRUIT AND SEED CRUNCH I call this a whole grain cookie—crunchy with a touch of sweet. Have one with a cup of tea when those latte-and-biscotti urges strike.

DOCTOR KRACKER (ALL FLATBREAD VARIETIES AND APPLE OAT CRUNCH CRISPS) Want some fun with a twist of gourmet? These totally taste like you're cheating! The seeds add both taste and a nutritional bonus. The Apple Cinnamon variety is an office favorite here at BNI, as it delivers the perfect combo of sweetness and crunch.

GG SCANDINAVIAN BRAN CRISPBREAD Okay, I confess: What you'll get here is sawdust and pure fiber. You must have hard-core weight-loss dedication to appreciate this one! But you can't beat the specs of 12 little calories and 5 grams of fiber per sheet. Tip: To make up for the plywood texture, pair it with something creamy, such as hummus, creamy goat cheese spread, or Laughing Cow Light.

MARY'S GONE CRACKERS ORIGINAL (WHEAT AND GLUTEN-FREE!) Although you should stick with larger flatbread crackers, these won't trap you into overeating because they're so hearty, and you get approximately ten for 100 calories. They don't look very appetizing, but tasting is believing—the combo of whole grain, brown rice, quinoa, flaxseed, and sesame seeds is yummy.

34 DEGREES WHOLE GRAIN CRISPBREAD The crackers are also smallish, but 18 of them will cost you only 70 calories.

Packaged Snacks

I'm willing to bet that America leads the world in packaged snacks. I swear I come across a new one every trip to the store. (If only we put this much ingenuity into developing a mascara that doesn't run!)

As you know, whole foods are always best, but there are so many times that call for packaged snacks: You're on the road, in an airport, at a friend's Super Bowl party—or you simply like keeping a few at home. So I've listed just a few packaged foods that are fun to eat and, yes, even *good* for you.

KIND BARS I'm cautious about the whole bar craze, particularly since some are glorified candy. KIND boasts that their products are "all natural whole nut and fruit bars made from ingredients you can see and pronounce." They're speaking my language! And they come in a bunch of flavors. Be sure to check the calories for the right fit—some are 175 and some 180, which is close enough for us to forgive, but no higher than 180, please!

GNU FLAVOR & FIBER BARS Start a Gnu routine with this brilliant on-the-go high fiber cereal alternative (see page 34) or snack option. It comes in a variety of flavors and it works when you're trapped at your desk, flying on a plane, or hiking the hills. The best part is that Gnu bars contain only about 130 calories and an awesome 12 grams of fiber. Tip: Freeze them to make them chewier, or warm them up like a pastry.

100-CALORIE PACKS OF NATURAL ALMONDS OR PISTACHIOS Want something better than a bar that contains nuts? How about just the nuts by themselves? Almonds are always a good option. And pistachios are my fave, because you get about thirty nuts for 100 calories (more than any other nut), and the shells keep you from plowing through them. That's why I refer to them as the skinny nut. Plus, these days they come in all kinds of flavors, like salt and pepper, chili lime, and garlic and onion.

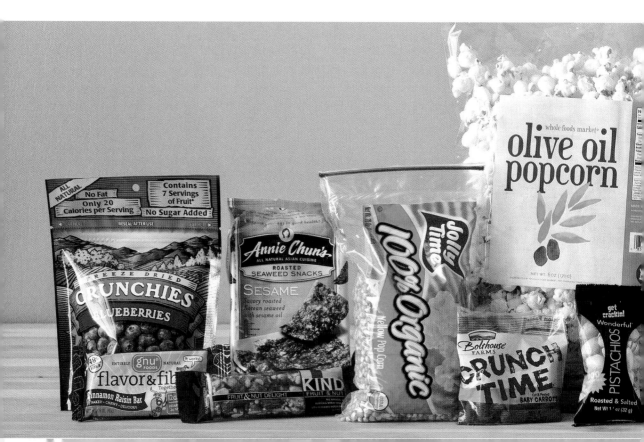

ORGANIC POPCORN KERNELS AND POPCORN I've already raved about popcorn—just thought I'd throw it in here as a reminder that popcorn is a winner. Buy brown paper lunch bags and microwave your own, without all the nasty add-on ingredients (see page 82).

BARNEY'S ALMOND BUTTER PACKS I was thrilled to find a 90-calorie single-serving pouch. (Who knows why 180 to 200 is the standard for nut butters?) With these packs, you can feel comfy about not overdoing it when you dip in. No guesswork!

PRESLICED, BAGGED APPLE SLICES You can find these in warehouse stores and supermarkets. Talk about a pure ingredient list! (Of course, to make it even better, look for one more word: organic.) Trust me, if you have them in your fridge or at work you *will* eat them, as they're refreshing, smart, and super-convenient.

TRADER JOE'S FIBER MINI CAKES/ZEN BAKERY FIBER CAKES The best thing about these cakes is that each one contains only 80 calories and delivers approximately 13 grams of fiber. If you can't find one near you, check out my recipe (see page 98). Tip: Be sure to refrigerate them; otherwise they'll turn green overnight since they have no preservatives.

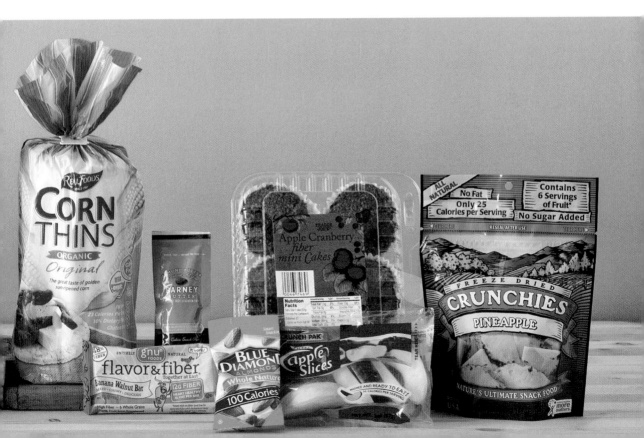

BABY CARROTS I know, you're probably accusing me of cheating here, since a bunch of veg in a bag doesn't count as a packaged snack, right? But baby carrots are convenient, colorful, and tasty, and they offer a satisfying crunch. And, oh yeah, they're healthy too. The junk food companies spend millions trying to come up with a snack this good!

CRUNCHIES BRAND FREEZE-DRIED FRUITS You know you've found a hit snack when kids approve of it! The pineapple tastes just like mini candy bites. Amazingly, these freeze-dried fruits retain much of the nutrient value of fresh fruit, so they're Rachel-approved too. They're a little pricey, so get them as a treat only when fresh fruit isn't practical. And keep your eye out—there are so many new brands popping up.

SEAWEED SNACKS Whoever imagined that Americans would want seaweed? But we do, and I'm all for it, since it's simple, low-cal, and packed with minerals. And there's no fishy flavor. Think potato chips without all the fat.

REAL FOODS ORGANIC CORN THINS A very simple packaged snack item—whole grain popped corn made into a corn cake. At just 23 calories per slice, this little number delivers big on taste and crunch. So many options for toppings (think hummus, goat cheese spread with sliced olives, honey mustard and turkey slices . . .)

the dairy case

Cheese

Many people say, "Are you kidding me?" when they find cheese as part of any nutrition plan. But the right kind of cheese in the right amount makes for a great snack or flavor enhancer. (Of course, I'm not talking "cheese foods" that come in a jar or spray can, which barely count as food.) Always think condiment-size (½ to 1 ounce). Picking up a big block of cheese will spell trouble. Buying individually sized and presliced is a must: That way you're automatically portion controlled. These are my go-to cheeses—they're convenient, small, and huge on taste.

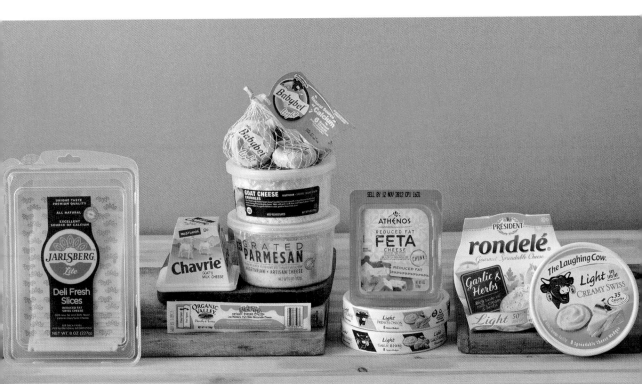

- Babybel Light
- Laughing Cow Light cheese wedge (buy a variety of flavors)
- Sliced Swiss cheese
- String cheese
- Creamy goat cheese (spread)
- Goat cheese (crumbled)
- Parmesan cheese
- Feta cheese
- Rondelé Light spreadable cheese

Milk Alternatives

I'm not totally against regular milk, but I prefer non-cow alternatives—and there are loads of them. Almost anything you choose is fine; what matters most is your taste preference. Just make sure to look for "unsweetened" and "fortified," with organic preferred! (See page 210 for more on organic dairy.)

- Almond
- Rice
- Coconut
- Soy
- Hemp

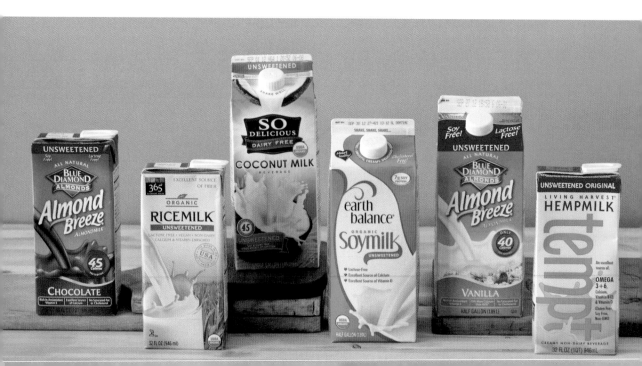

Yogurt

Here are my guidelines on what to grab:

CHOOSE GREEK OR GOAT YOGURT, BUT SKIP THE FLAVORED VARIETIES (less protein, much, much, *much* more sugar)—and stick with nonfat plain. Then add fruit, cinnamon, and a touch of my recommended jam, apple butter (see page 195), or any other natural sweetener, such as honey.

LOOK AT THE END OF THE INGREDIENTS LIST: If you see "live and active cultures," that's good—but no guarantee they'll survive the digestive tract. Seek cultures that are also probiotics (not all are), such as *Lactobacillus acidophilus, Bifidus regularis*, and *L.casei*. They can survive the journey to improve digestive health. Also be on the lookout for the "Live Active Culture" seal that makes picking one out easy, since it means the yogurt contains enough active bacteria to get the job done.

All of these brands—Chobani, Fage, Oikos, and Brown Cow—fit those guidelines.

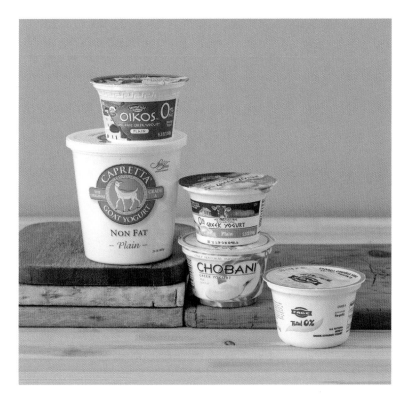

dressings, oils, and condiments (oh my!)

Here's a quick snapshot of my go-to pantry oils and dressings.

Dressings

Oil and vinegar are the best choices for dressing (no added ingredients—just pure and simple). But if you want to shake things up once in a while, go for a bottled variety with a simple, short ingredients list, and be mindful of the sodium content. Here are the few I recommend:

GALEOS The natural ingredients list—and hint of pure miso—really raises the bar on the average dressing. It's low in sodium, and there are so many flavors to try. Be sure to look out for the individual to-go packets. Toss one of these in your bag and save serious calories next time you're dining out!

BOLTHOUSE OLIVE OIL AND YOGURT-BASED DRESSINGS An olive oil–based bottled dressing is always a plus—and the yogurt-based versions are a one-package combo of creamy and flavorful, with smart nutritional specs. There are lots of flavors to choose from that contain just 45 calories or less in 2 tablespoons. In addition to salads, these dressings are great as a marinade. I also like that they can be found in most markets (in the refrigerated section of the produce department).

NEWMAN'S OWN LITE Although slightly higher in sodium than Bolthouse and Galeos, these are also about 45 calories per 2 tablespoons and are available at almost any grocery store. There are many varieties, but Sesame Ginger and Lite Balsamic are favorites with my patients.

BASIC SALAD DRESSING RULES

Can't find any of my picks? Just follow these simple guidelines:

- Keep one serving (usually 2 tablespoons) to 80 calories or less.

- Don't buy fat-free—you want *some* fat for nutrient absorption.

- Choose one that includes high-quality oils like olive oil—my favorite.

- Avoid a huge laundry list of ingredients. Think simple—more ingredients usually means more additives and preservatives.

- Look out for sodium: If the Daily Value is greater than 20%, it is too high.

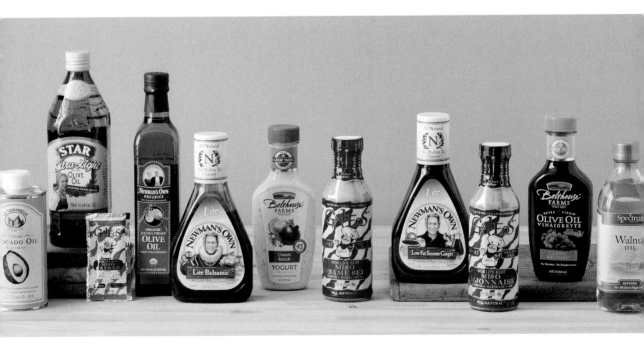

COOL DARK PLACES AREN'T ONLY FOR CELEBRITIES— THAT'S WHERE YOU STORE YOUR OIL!

It's not just the *Twilight* characters who avoid harsh light. The same goes for your cooking oils. Even if stored under perfect conditions, many oils degrade entirely after only twelve months, losing flavor and nutrients. So follow these rules:

- Don't buy more oil than you'll use in six months.
- Store oil in a cool, dark place, or refrigerate after opening.
- Buy oils in tinted glass to protect against light exposure.
- Pick bottles from the back of the shelf—again, less exposure to light.

Oils

When it comes to oils, my top pick for almost everything is olive oil. But there's more to know about choosing the right olive oil for the job. Each has different smoke points, and that matters for your health (see page 227).

EXTRA VIRGIN OLIVE OIL (UNREFINED COLD PRESSED) This super-high-quality oil has a low smoke point (320 degrees), so it's best reserved for salads and cold dishes. It has a nice strong flavor and greenish tint from the chlorophyll pigments.

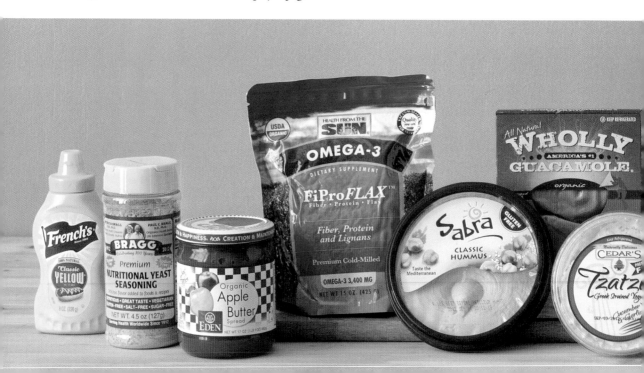

EXTRA VIRGIN OLIVE OIL (REFINED) With a smoke point of 406 degrees, this variety is what you want for high to medium-heat cooking, such as baking, braising, or a gentle sauté.

EXTRA LIGHT OLIVE OIL This olive oil has the highest smoke point (468 degrees). Reach for it when doing any high-heat cooking, like broiling, grilling, stir-frying, and roasting. And it has a neutral taste, so it won't affect the flavor of your dish. P.S.: The word "light" refers to the olive oil's color, fragrance, and taste—*not* fat or calories.

AVOCADO OIL It's pricey, but worth treating yourself to! It adds a soft, buttery taste and a mild avocado aroma to salads—and because it has a high smoke point (520 degrees), it can be used for high-heat cooking like stir-frying and searing. And it's rich in monounsaturated fats.

WALNUT OIL Also a bit more expensive than olive oil, but incredibly flavorful and delicious. It's got a nutty taste and aroma and, like the nut it came from, it's rich in omega-3 fats. With a smoke point of 400°F, it's good for sautéing and pan-frying. It really shines in cold dishes, though.

Condiments and Toppings

Move aside, ketchup: It's time for a whole new approach to add-ons. It's no longer enough that they taste good—they have to *do* good, too! I've listed my must-have condiments and toppings. Some can be dashed atop finished dishes, others are for cooking only. The fun part is experimenting until you discover what you like best. With all condiments, watch the sodium and sugar.

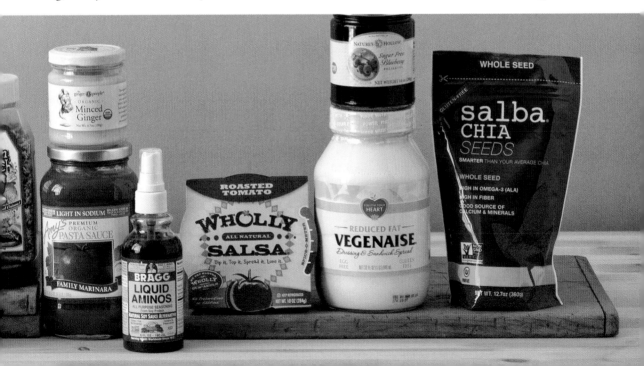

WHITE CHIA (SALBA CHIA PREFERRED) My absolute ultimate favorite fiber, antioxidant, and omega-3 booster! It has a neutral taste, and I insist on the white chia, as dark chia's charcoal color looks like scrapings off an oven wall (and when it comes to creating good eating habits, looks matter). There are two chia options: whole seeds and ground. Most of my patients prefer the whole seeds, as the ground kind changes the texture of your food.

GROUND FLAXSEED Rich in protective omega-3s and lignans, its taste isn't as neutral as chia, and you need to grind it in a coffee grinder or buy it ground to score the benefits. Keep in mind that once opened, ground flaxseed deteriorates after 45 to 60 days, so make sure it's vacuum-packed, and refrigerate it in an airtight container. My absolute fave is FiPro Flax.

SALSA It's the most popular condiment in America today—even more so than ketchup. And good thing, too, because all those great ingredients provide so much flavor and nutrition for a mere 10 calories (about 2 tablespoons). Salsa's benefits come primarily from the lycopene in the tomatoes. If you can handle hot and spicy, you'll score additional benefits, as chile peppers contain capsaicin, which may also help boost metabolism.

FRENCH'S MUSTARD Okay, I know, you're wondering how this 'ol American standard got featured as a "nutritional winner." It just seems so . . . basic. Well, you know that trademark bright yellow color? That comes from turmeric, one of my favorite spices because of its known anti-inflammatory properties. And any opportunity to add a touch of turmeric to your diet is a great nutritional move!

TZATZIKI Tzatziki is a thick, tangy Greek yogurt dip that's filled with garlic, cucumber, olive oil, and sometimes lemon juice and dill. It tastes amazing spooned onto pita bread, salads, and other Mediterranean specialties. At 35 calories per 2 tablespoons, it's a creamy keeper! Find it in the refrigerated section of the market near the hummus.

MINCED GINGER (ANY BRAND) Keep a jar of this exotic and spicy root within reach in your fridge to add a kick—and some anti-inflammatory benefits—to any dish.

BRAGG NUTRITIONAL YEAST Flavor and nutrition in one shot! No salt, no sugar—and we're talking only 20 calories per tablespoon—yet it packs an amazing cheese-like flavor. Plus, it's loaded with vitamin B_{12}, making it one of the best energy foods around. Add it to soups, Greek yogurt dips, pasta, and popcorn.

BRAGG LIQUID AMINOS Want to take the boring out of steamed veg? Impossible? Then you haven't tried liquid aminos. Similar in taste to soy sauce, but different in that the salty taste comes from naturally occurring sodium found in soybeans without added table salt or preservatives. Buy the kind in the spray bottle to keep the sodium under control. It adds a flavor boost to anything.

MARINARA Low-sodium marinara sauce adds flavor and a hefty shot of lycopene to any meal. I use this a lot. Stock up!

HUMMUS It's not just a dip. Mix it with lemon juice to make a yummy salad dressing, or even a topping for rice. These days, you'll also find numerous flavors so you'll never tire of it.

FOLLOW YOUR HEART REDUCED-FAT VEGENAISE Say good-bye to full-fat mayo forever. This vegan (egg-free) spread tastes just like real mayo, and makes a perfect substitute, particularly for your Sunday Salads. A little pricey but worth a try.

WHOLLY GUACAMOLE (ANY VARIETY) You've probably seen avocados advertised as a superfood. This handy guac comes readymade in a pouch. There are even 100-calorie packs, which make for a perfect portable snack when paired with baby carrots. Love that Wholly Guacamole is an easy find—usually next to the hummus.

LOEB'S ONION CRUNCH You know those overly processed, crunchy, onion-like things that people fling atop green beans at Thanksgiving? Get to unknow them. Instead, get to know Loeb's Onion Crunch: just 35 cal for 2 tablespoons, and it makes a fun accessory to soups, veg, anything—and particularly boring Thanksgiving dishes.

NATURE'S HOLLOW JAMS Among my patients, Nature's Hollow jams win every taste test—they love it in plain Greek yogurt. They're naturally sweetened with xylitol, which has a very low glycemic index and fewer calories than regular jams. But moderation is still key! Spot it at your local health food store or order online.

EDEN'S APPLE BUTTER SPREAD Love apple butter! This one is not only organic but also low-cal. Simplicity at its best: It's just apples that have been simmered with a touch of apple juice—and nothing else. Swirl it into oatmeal or yogurt, or spread onto toast. One tablespoon is all you need!

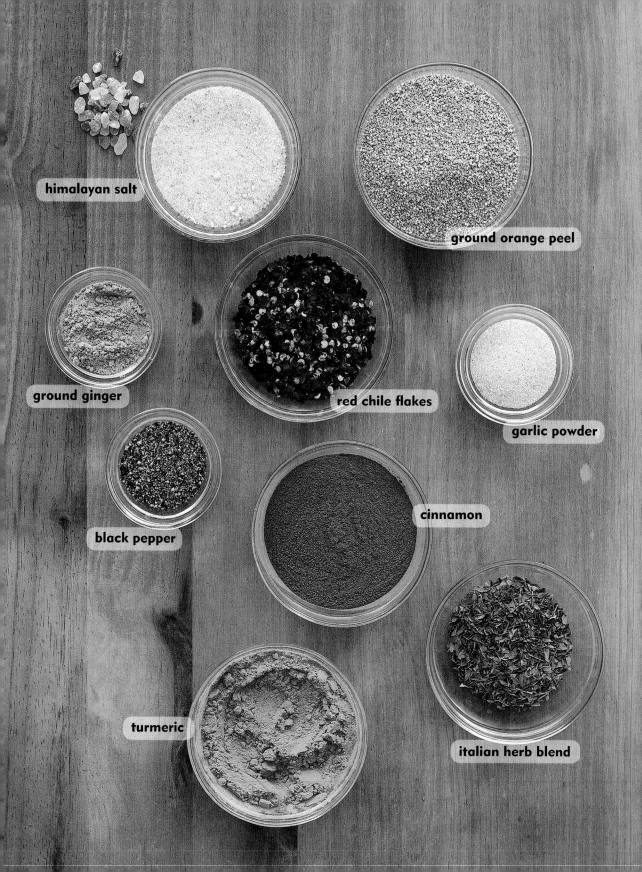

himalayan salt

ground orange peel

ground ginger

red chile flakes

garlic powder

black pepper

cinnamon

turmeric

italian herb blend

pantry essentials

Dried Herbs, Spices, and More

Spices and herbs do *way* more than make food taste better. Just a few sprinkles can deliver such powerful health boosts that no dish should go without 'em! That's why I created entire spice mixes (see pages 28 and 40).

Now, you'd need a whole room to store all the spices and herbs available today, so I narrowed this list down to my pantry faves, including those spices used in my special shakers and recipes.

- Cinnamon (Ceylon preferred)
- Turmeric
- Garlic powder
- Ground ginger
- Ground orange peel (organic)
- Italian herb blend (oregano, basil, thyme)
- Red chile flakes
- Black pepper
- Himalayan salt (great mineral content compared to table salt)

sweeteners

We all know the cycle. You eat something sweet, and then you want more, and more, and it doesn't stop!

How do you avoid this? Three tips: moderation, moderation, and more moderation. The more you indulge in sugar, the more your body wants. But if you train your taste buds that "a little is enough," they eventually learn to obey.

So when you do need a touch of sweetness, try some of these options.

BLACKSTRAP MOLASSES This sweetener contains minerals that promote health, including calcium, potassium, and iron. With 32 little calories in 2 teaspoons, it's a great sweetener for tea, oatmeal, and baked goods. Tip: Look for *unsulphured* and preferably organic. Store it in a cool, dark place.

STEVIA PACKS OR STEVIA VANILLA DROPS Although stevia contains zero calories, it's *intensely* sweet, so go easy with it. The best use: Add a few drops to plain Greek yogurt. Depending on the part of the plant a particular stevia product comes from, it may have a slightly bitter or very sweet aftertaste. There are many brands, but I prefer NuStevia. (Easily found online.)

HONEY Just like with chocolate, the darker the better! Darker honeys contain more vitamins and trace minerals than lighter ones. And a teaspoon comes in with a mere 22 calories.

SUCANAT Sucanat tastes like brown sugar but is less processed (the name comes from "sugar cane natural"). Because it's not heavily refined, it retains its nutrient-rich molasses and minerals such as iron, calcium, and potassium. At just 15 calories per teaspoon, it's a practical sugar alternative.

RAW AGAVE Raw agave is less processed (which explains its darker color) than regular agave, and it's much sweeter, so you'll need less of it. Agave has about 20 calories per teaspoon.

COCONUT PALM SUGAR Not only does this taste a bit like caramel (yum!), it's gentler on your blood sugar levels than sucrose—and it contains amino acids, minerals, and B vitamins. But that doesn't mean go to town with it! Stick with 1 teaspoon, which adds 18 calories.

PURE MAPLE SYRUP Betcha didn't know that grade B syrup is a smarter choice than grade A. Why? Grade B is thicker and delivers a stronger maple flavor, so just a little bit does a big job on the flavor front. And that means you won't need to use loads of it; just 1 teaspoon comes in with about 17 calories.

JOSEPH'S SUGAR FREE SYRUP Sweetened with maltitol, this is a favorite of my diabetic patients. It tastes great, especially compared to the other "healthy syrup" options in health food stores. The only drawback: Some people are sensitive to maltitol, which is a sugar alcohol that can cause bloating (although I have yet to hear any complaints from my patients). Just 3 little calories per teaspoon!

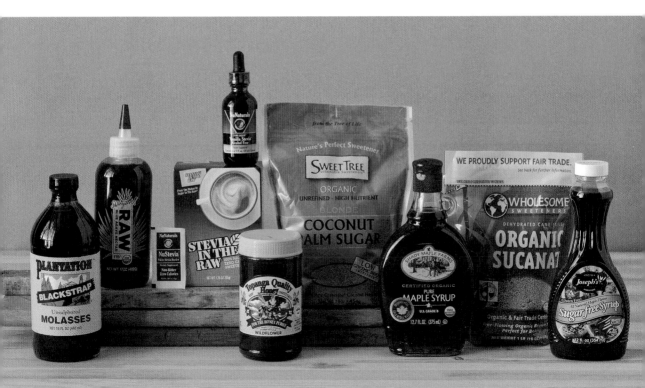

sweet treats

We all have one, and it can be very demanding—forcing us to do things we regret later. I'm referring to the sweet tooth, of course. Sure, we can keep it calm with kinda-sorta treats, like my breakfast parfaits. But sometimes it just insists on bites of pure sweetness. And we all know if you don't address it, it will come back and hit you in the a** and hips (literally).

So I came up with a few treats without the tricks here, just pure fun—and some of them even offer up health benefits which truly make them worth every bite. (One word for you: *chocolate*.)

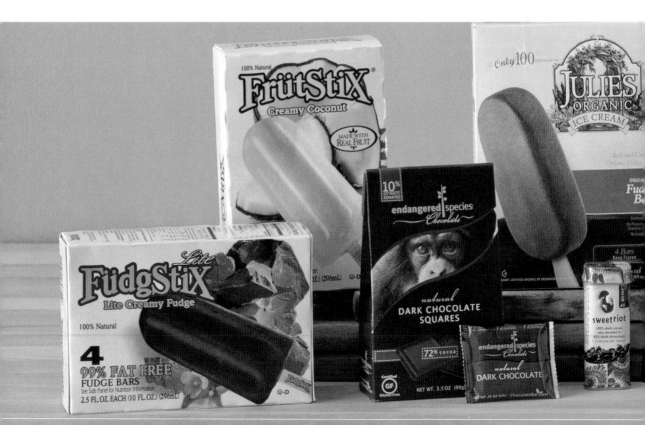

SWEET RIOT CACAO NIBS These nibs are dark chocolate–covered cacao bits that come in a pocket-sized tin. Each piece has just 1 to 2 calories, making them an *amazing* chocolate-craving solution. The 100 percent cacao beans in the center are the real deal, loaded with a ton of antioxidants (more than red wine) and heart-healthy flavanols, with the dark chocolate coating sealing the deal. Warning: These can be addictive!

GHIRARDELLI OR ENDANGERED SPECIES CHOCOLATE SQUARES Did I mention that I love chocolate? At BNI, I prescribe an ounce or two of 70 percent dark chocolate several times per week, and these perfectly fill the prescription. In each box you'll find individually wrapped 50- to 55-calorie 70 percent dark chocolate squares. They're not "Dutch processed" (a treatment that results in a milder taste but also strips out a lot of the antioxidants). They also contain little sugar, and the preportioned squares will keep you in check at snack time.

FRUTSTIX, JULIE'S ORGANIC, AND SKINNY COW FROZEN TREATS This is for when you didn't have time to make your own dessert (see page 84) and you know that ice cream tub will set your diet back a few centuries. What do you do? Try one—and just *one*—of these frozen fudge or sorbet-type bars. The rule is that they must be premeasured on a stick, with simple ingredients, low calories, and no high-fructose corn syrup or artificial sweeteners. (If you can't find these specific varieties, don't just trust the brand; look at the ingredients list.)

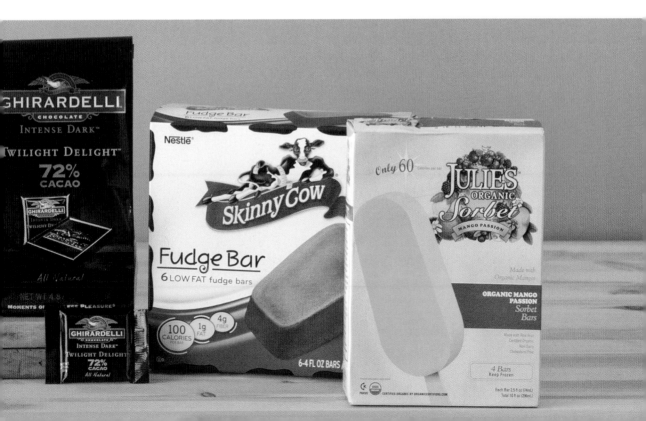

must-have
kitchen accessories

Want to build a solid foundation? Then you need the right tools! I stock my kitchen with the following items. They make cooking easier and healthier—and none of 'em will break the bank. In fact, some will even help you save money!

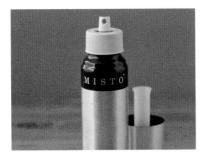

MISTO SPRAYER This nonaerosol, propellant- and chemical-free oil sprayer will give you just the right amount of oil. It's also more cost-effective than other nonstick sprays, because you fill it with your own oil. Tip: Fill with olive oil and vinegar and mist your salad.

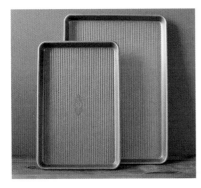

BAKING SHEET/COOKIE SHEET This must-have will make roasting veg, fish—practically anything—easy. No need to spray if you use parchment paper. It's worth picking up full and half sheet pans.

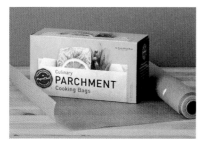

PARCHMENT PAPER AND BAGS Total cleanup—and calorie—saver! Just line your baking sheet with parchment paper or simply use one of the bags and toss after cooking. And they save you from needing to oil the baking sheet to keep food from sticking (which can bake on and ruin it, anyway).

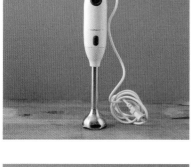

IMMERSION BLENDER Regular blenders are a pain to clean, particularly if you're mixing multiple items (such as smoothies, fro-yo, and soups). With the stick, just rinse the tip and you're ready to whiz up the next item.

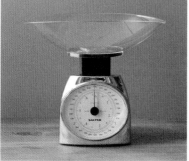

FOOD SCALE Everyone has a bathroom scale, but most people don't have a scale where it matters first: in the kitchen! A good scale provides your portion control reality check. During the first few weeks, use it as a training tool to help you learn what a serving of protein looks like at a glance (a skill you'll need in restaurants). Once you've mastered estimating portions, don't tuck the scale too far away—you'll need it to occasionally remind you how much is enough.

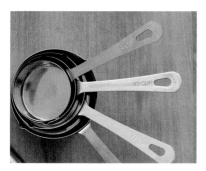

MEASURING CUPS AND MEASURING SPOONS The difference between a tablespoon and a teaspoon can make a big difference in your diet. Same with measuring cups—especially when it comes to cereal or grains like brown rice. Tip: Leave a ½ or 1 cup spoon measuring cup in your cereal box so you don't go overboard.

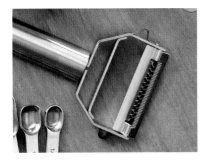

JULIENNE PEELER This simple, inexpensive tool comes in handy for making my amazing zucchini "spaghetti" (see page 146 for the recipe).

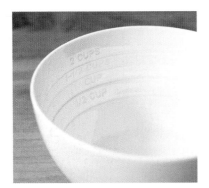

MEASURE-UP BOWL Talk about convenience. This bowl means no more guesstimating your portions—just pour to the line and you're good to go. You can't get it wrong!

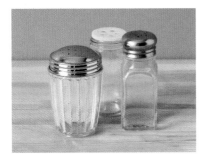

EMPTY SHAKERS Fill 'em up with my special spice mixes—the Shaker Waker-Upper (page 28) and Magical Mystery Mix (page 40).

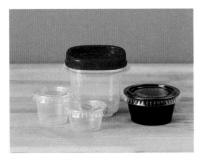

TO-GO DRESSING CONTAINERS Super-handy to help keep portions in check when it comes to nut butters and dressings (see page 77). You can find them online or at restaurant supply stores.

just the facts

THE SCIENCE BEHIND THE SECRETS

Why?

That's the second most common question I hear at the office—the first being "What do I do?"

Some patients follow whatever action plan I recommend, no questions. ("Rachel, just tell me what to eat!") But many want to know the science behind my recommendations. It helps them stick to the plan and explain it to their friends and family, who can then provide moral support—or, better yet, join them.

Knowing the science also helps them cut through the hype. Here in the United States, we're surrounded by thousands of foods and supplements making all sorts of health claims—many of which aren't confirmed or even approved by the FDA. That's why so many people jump at products or programs that lack nutritional fundamentals, such as weight-loss plans that leave them starving for nutrients, or organic vegan options that make them overweight.

They need the science, and I'm more than happy to provide it!

Working as a nutrition researcher in cancer institutes and hospitals, I became well-versed in how to incorporate clinical research into the patient setting. A few years later, I started Beller Nutritional Institute to translate all that science into an accessible format that my patients could understand and appreciate.

So instead of writing two books—one offering nutrition advice with scientific notations, the other providing a fun-filled action plan—I decided to do what I do at the office: put it all together. After all, delicious should always go with nutritious!

You saw my secrets and recommendations in the action-oriented first part of this book. Now for the research. But don't fear: I've written it so it's easy to swallow.

the science behind the f-word

Your Fiber-Rich Breakfast: Where Did the Magic Numbers Come From?

The magic numbers—30 to 35 grams of fiber daily for women, 35 to 40 grams for men—are not arbitrary. I derived them from scientific studies. And the vast majority agree: For both weight loss and better health, you should make fiber a foundation of your diet.

Unfortunately, most Americans average just 11 to 15 grams of fiber on their "good days."[1] So here are some amazing reasons to increase your fiber intake:

Fiber Makes Weight Loss Easier

So many companies claim they've got an easy weight-loss solution. Well, maybe it's time to put away the infomercial gadgets and questionable fat-burning pills. Study after study points to fiber as a key weight-loss weapon.

Fiber supports weight loss in so many ways. First, high-fiber foods tend to have fewer calories. Second, fiber extends the length of time a hormone called cholecystokinin (CCK) tells your brain that you're full. Third, fiber takes up significant space in your stomach, so you'll be less likely to overeat—especially if you start every single day with a high-fiber breakfast.

The fourth reason is really interesting: Fiber may actually remove excess calories from your body before they can be absorbed. A study by the University of Kiel in Germany found that every gram of fiber eaten removes 7 calories,[2] so eating 35 grams of fiber a day could knock about 245 calories off your daily intake! While more research needs to be done in this area, if the Kiel scientists' work is true, *you could lose a half a pound a week just by eating more fiber.*

Fiber Boosts Your Heart Health

Remember when I told you about the cleansing effects of fiber? Researchers have found that reason: Soluble fibers grab onto cholesterol and prevents its reabsorption by your body.

In addition, several large studies have found that *in*soluble fibers lower heart disease risk—perhaps because the whole grains that contain insoluble fibers pack other beneficial compounds, such as lignans, antioxidants, and phytoestrogens, which may reduce inflammation, blood pressure, and the risk of blood clots.[3]

Fiber Reduces Your Risk of Diabetes

The reports are in: Not just one, but two large studies found that people whose diets contained the most fiber from grains (insoluble fibers) had a 35 percent lower incidence of type 2 diabetes.

In addition, soluble fiber from oats and barley moderates blood sugar levels by slowing the absorption of carbohydrates.

And a high-fiber diet has also been shown to help those who are already suffering from the disease. In one study, when insulin-resistant women's intake of insoluble fiber was increased, their intestinal bacteria seemed to change after about 6 months on a high-fiber diet—and they became more responsive to insulin.[4] So it pays to stick it out to give fiber a fighting chance.

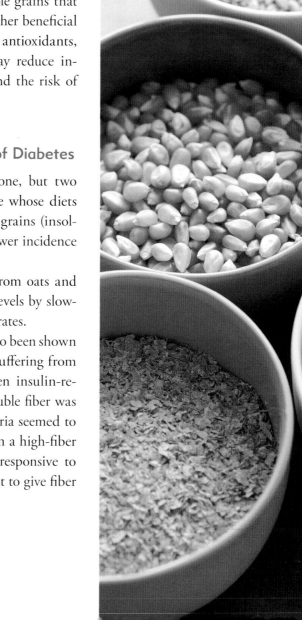

Fiber Lowers Your Odds of Getting Breast Cancer

Studies continue to show a link between eating fiber and a reduction in breast cancer risk. One way insoluble fiber does this is by sticking to free estrogens in the gut and sweeping them out.[5] Researchers believe fiber may also ensure that less estrogen is free in the first place.

What do I mean by "free"? Typically estrogen—which is tied up in food—reaches the stomach and is separated and freed up for absorption by intestinal bacteria. But studies have found that when women eat a diet rich in fiber (and low in fat), their intestinal bacteria actually becomes less efficient at freeing up estrogen. The upshot: Less estrogen is absorbed and you end up exposed to lower amounts of the hormone, which in turn is what may reduce your risk of breast cancer.[6]

That could be why women who have a high-fiber diet have a lower incidence of breast cancer. The Swedish Mammography Cohort found that high-fiber diets translated into 15 percent lower risk of breast cancer. And evidence from the famed Harvard Nurses' Health Study, which followed approximately 88,000 women for eighteen years, suggests that getting 30 grams of fiber daily gives you the *maximum* risk reduction for breast cancer. Women who consumed 30 grams a day had a whopping 32 percent decreased risk. By comparison, the women in the study who ate less than 25 grams a day only had a 2 percent reduction. To me, that's a clear case for eating your Daily 35![7]

And then there's one more big benefit worth touting here . . .

Fiber Helps You Live Longer

Here's the math: The 2012 European Prospective Investigation into Cancer and Nutrition examined the diets of 450,000 men and women. Those who ate the most high-fiber foods—vegetables, fruits, beans, and whole grains—tended to live longer. Every 10 grams of fiber per day cut overall mortality risk by 10 percent—and cut the risk of dying specifically from digestive diseases by nearly 40 percent.[8]

(And not only does fiber reduce mortality, it appears to increase lifespan.) In other words, the secret to long life just might be found in natural high-fiber foods.

A landmark study led by the National Cancer Institute linked fiber with dramatic boosts to longevity. High-fiber diets also reduced the incidence of death from cancers (including those of the head and neck, esophagus, liver, bladder, and kidney) as well as from cardiovascular disease.[9] Although researchers don't know exactly how fiber protects us from these diseases, these studies clearly show the value of making fiber a long-term priority.[10]

Keep It Real: The Truth Behind Isolated Fibers

Not all fibers are created equal. Food manufacturers have developed what they call "functional fibers," which are isolated or extracted from whole grains and added to our foods.

Now, in order to be defined as a functional fiber, these additives must benefit our health. One such functional fiber you may have heard of is psyllium—which is extracted from psyllium seed husks and used in Metamucil and other products. Psyllium not only increases total fiber content, but it also may decrease total blood cholesterol and LDL cholesterol. Therefore, it can be called a functional fiber. Oat and barley beta glucans are other functional fibers with proven benefits.

However, the scientific jury is still out on manufactured *isolated* fibers. Many health professionals question whether they're as effective at keeping you full,[11] lowering cholesterol, managing glucose levels, and providing the same benefits as true whole food (nonmanufactured) fibers. Furthermore, many question whether to include isolated fibers in the total fiber count on food labels. So, until the research is conclusive, I strongly recommend that you get your fiber fix from *whole foods* (whole grains, fruits, and vegetables) and don't rely on manufactured isolated fibers.

It All Adds Up: Get Your Fiber Fix

Yes, there's much more to learn about fiber. That's why scientists continue to conduct studies—and will never state that anything is "100 percent conclusive." (After all, we used to know that we had nine planets in our solar system, but as our knowledge continued to evolve, we came to realize that there actually are only eight—poor Pluto!)

Yet while there's more to learn, there's still much to *love*.

Of course, fiber rarely works alone: Most of us don't just eat whole wheat for breakfast. Those who have cereal usually enjoy it with cow's milk or yogurt, so I've decided to also include the latest science on dairy products.

The Lowdown on Dairy

We Americans love our dairy products—and are constantly finding new ways to consume it. I mean, how many different kinds of lattes can there be?

Yet almost every day, a patient asks me whether he or she should eat dairy products. It's a hot topic that gets a lot of media attention—and rightfully so, because the findings are quite conflicting.

On one hand, cow's milk provides vitamin D, calcium, protein, and a compound called conjugated linoleic acid (CLA), which has been shown to fight tumor growth in cells and laboratory animals.[12]

But cow's milk can also contain unwanted fat and hormones, so you must carefully select the types of dairy you consume. Unless you're lactose intolerant, you don't need to swear off dairy entirely—my motto is everything in moderation—but you should follow these guidelines to make informed decisions.

The Skinny on Skim

My basic rule when it comes to dairy: choose low-fat or, ideally, no-fat. A lot of research shows that a low-fat diet reduces cancer risk; unfortunately, many dairy products are high in fat (think cheese and ice cream).

Drinking organic nonfat milk also minimizes the hormones. That said, milk naturally has hormones, and no solid conclusions have been drawn about their possible effects. (See the details in the next section.)

The possible downside to skim: It contains added milk solids to restore the protein and calcium lost during the fat-removal process. Some believe these milk solids produce oxidized cholesterol that can damage arteries, but the amount of oxidized cholesterol in skim milk is so small that I wouldn't worry about it.

If you're still concerned, then limit your intake or forget skim and choose a dairy alternative such as soy, almond, or coconut milk. I'll talk more about these in a few pages.
My recommendation? As I say again and again: everything in moderation.

Watch Out for Extra Hormones

Everyone knows hormones are a fundamental part of life. The hormones our bodies naturally produce help us digest food, grow, develop, reproduce, and even shape our moods.

What keeps us researchers up late studying and debating are *food*-based hormones. You've probably seen milk with labels that boast "no added hormones." The truth is that *all* milk from animals (including humans) contains natural growth hormones and estrogens. After all, that's what helps babies grow!

Unfortunately, some types of milk contain *extra* estrogens. This includes milk from cows treated with synthetic hormones, such as recombinant bovine growth hormone (rBGH) and a

For those who feared that all this science would take the joy out of eating, take a look at one sampling of a breakfast that comes from all these findings:

- A bowl of nonfat Greek yogurt topped with high-fiber cereal and cinnamon
- A cup of matcha tea with lemon juice

You get protein, calcium, antioxidants, and a dose of fiber that can whisk away hormones, excess cholesterol, and other things you don't want. In addition, these ingredients combine to regulate your blood sugar, which research suggests is a key strategy for disease prevention.

Best of all, this breakfast combo is easy and totally tasty.

milk-producing hormone called bST. High levels of estrogens are also found in cows kept in a pregnant-like state three hundred days a year to increase their milk production.

To avoid these extra hormones, drink organic milk from cows not treated with hormones. As a nutritional bonus, a study in the *Journal of the Science of Food and Agriculture* found that organic milk contained 67 percent more antioxidants and vitamins compared to conventional milk, and more of the beneficial fats, including 39 percent more omega-3 fatty acids and 60 percent more CLA fatty acid.[13] For years the question of whether or not organic milk is more nutritious than conventional milk has been debated. Technically, they have the same amount of total fat and protein. However, as I just mentioned, the added bonus of antioxidants and vitamins and the *type* of fat in organic milk tips the scale in favor of organic over conventional.

Organic milk still contains natural growth hormones. In fact, research from the FDA shows only a tiny difference between conventional and organic milk when it comes to the hormone IGF-1.[14] And that's where the discussion gets really heated.

Get Smart About: Insulin-like Growth Factor (IGF-1)

IGF-1 sounds like something from a science-fiction novel. Indeed, when it comes to this natural compound, scientists are still working to separate the facts from the fiction.

Our bodies naturally produce IGF-1, which, among other things, helps the body absorb and use calcium. However, IGF-1 also helps tumors grow, and some research links high levels of IGF-1 in the blood to an increased risk of hormone-sensitive tumors, such as breast and ovarian cancer in women and testicular cancer in men.[15]

Researchers in the United States and France (where people eat a lot of high-fat dairy) have found a moderate relationship between milk consumption and increased levels of IGF-1 in human blood.[16] However, pasteurization and digestion both break down IGF-1 in milk, so scientists don't know exactly where that extra IGF-1 comes from. Since we don't absorb IGF-1 from foods, something in milk may stimulate our own bodies to produce extra IGF-1.

Now, don't panic about IGF-1.

Keep in mind that your body produces more IGF-1 from your saliva and digestive tract than you get from food sources, and that IGF-1 has many useful functions. Also know that scientists have not found a conclusive link between eating dairy and an increased risk of cancer.[17] The Harvard Nurses' Health Study actually found that for premenopausal women, consuming low-fat dairy reduced the risk of breast cancer.[18] (I told you this topic was complicated!)

As always, I stress moderation. Until researchers determine the specific role IGF-1 plays in tumor growth, it makes sense to go easy on milk, especially if you're at an increased risk for developing a hormone-sensitive cancer.

(As a bonus, reducing your IGF-1 intake might have a beauty benefit: Dermatologists suspect that IGF-1 stimulation could cause acne.[19])

Need a good milk alternative? Then . . .

Go Greek!

You can't toss a spoon in a supermarket without it landing in some Greek yogurt product—everything from dips to ice cream have hopped on the bandwagon.

And that's because the benefits of Greek yogurt keep piling up: You get more protein per spoonful than in regular yogurt, not to mention all the live and active cultures and probiotics to promote good digestion. *And* you don't have to worry as much about IGF-1.

A 2002 study published in *Cancer Epidemiology, Biomarkers & Prevention* found that eating yogurt did *not* increase IGF-1 levels in the body. Scientists believe that IGF-1 could be inactivated during the process of turning milk into yogurt.[20]

The bottom line: Your best dairy source is nonfat organic Greek yogurt.

Of course, most people still need a *liquid* option. As much as I love Greek yogurt, I wouldn't recommend it in your coffee! Fortunately, there are options.

What to Know About Milk Alternatives—and Other A.M. Beverages

Cow's milk has lost its monopoly. Today you'll find many nondairy milk options: almond, rice, soy, even hemp milk. Since they are all plant-based, you don't have to worry about cholesterol, added hormones (or the ethics of animal-sourced foods), or IGF-1. And many come unsweetened and fortified with calcium and vitamin D— which are pluses from both weight and health perspectives.

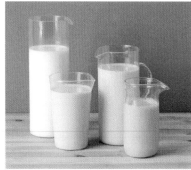

Of course, you can add these alternatives to coffee, but I'd like to recommend one more morning beverage alternative: Instead of coffee, drink black tea—or, my ultimate favorite, high-quality matcha green tea. Both provide caffeine but also contain the antioxidant epigallocatechin gallate, or EGCG, which emerging research suggests may decrease your risk for inflammatory diseases such as diabetes, heart disease, and certain cancers.

The best part is that matcha contains *three times* more EGCG than other green teas.[21] When you steep tea bags or loose teas, only 5 to 10 percent of the nutrients end up in the cup because most are not water-soluble. Most of the minerals, vitamins, and antioxidants are literally thrown out with the tea leaves. With matcha, the whole tea leaf is ground into a fine powder and consumed entirely—so you get 100 percent of the nutrients from the leaves.

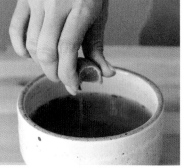

The perfect breakfast drink: matcha plus a splash of citrus = an antioxidant-rich alarm clock.

Want nutrition bonus points? Add a splash of citrus such as lemon, lime, or O.J. to your tea. Studies show citrus maximizes your absorption of EGCG and significantly increases its antioxidant value.

the science behind the flip-it method

It All Begins with Veggies—and Here's Why

You know how some doctors talk about "Recommended Daily Allowance"? Well, when it comes to vegetables, I can't say enough—and you can't *have* enough. Why? (And no, it's not because I own a farm—I eat plants, I don't grow them.) It's because of my background in oncological nutrition: During all those years of intensive research, I came across overwhelming evidence that a vegetable-rich diet is your smartest move, whether you're trying to lose weight or prevent disease. That's what led me to develop the Flip-It Method (see pages 36 to 40). Let's look at the benefits for each one:

Veggies Support Weight Loss

It seems like all we ever hear about are fad diets: cleanse this, eliminate that. The scary part? Many of them have no scientific basis whatsoever. Some celebrity or wannabe expert latches onto something, hires a great marketer, and away we go.

If all the hard research linking veg consumption to a healthier weight was promoted the way fad diets are, everyone would be devouring kale and zucchini by the acre. It may sound simplistic (shouldn't getting skinny involve complicated rules and cutting tasty foods?), but the facts don't lie. One study at Beth Israel Deaconess Medical Center, for example, looked at the habits that successful weight losers share. Many of them had to do with the tried-and-true advice to eat healthier and get more exercise. The stats: 41 percent switched to foods like veggies that have fewer calories, and 44 percent ate less fat (something most veggies don't have, of course). The researchers also discovered what *didn't* work or *didn't* last were faddish diets, over-the-counter diet pills, and diet foods.[22]

How do vegetables help with weight loss? For starters, they're naturally low-cal and contain fiber. But there's also good evidence that veggies add so much *volume* to your diet—at such a small caloric cost—that you slim down while still feeling satisfied. Hard to believe? Well, get this: Pennsylvania State University researchers found that men and women on produce-heavy

BETCHA DIDN'T KNOW: Some like it hot. You've heard the hype about raw food diets, but tomatoes are actually healthier cooked than raw. Heat releases the antioxidant lycopene from the tomato's fibers—and if you add a touch of oil (such as olive oil) during cooking, your body will absorb more of those cancer-fighting compounds. That's why you'll find tomatoes in many of my meal suggestions. The secret really is in the sauce!

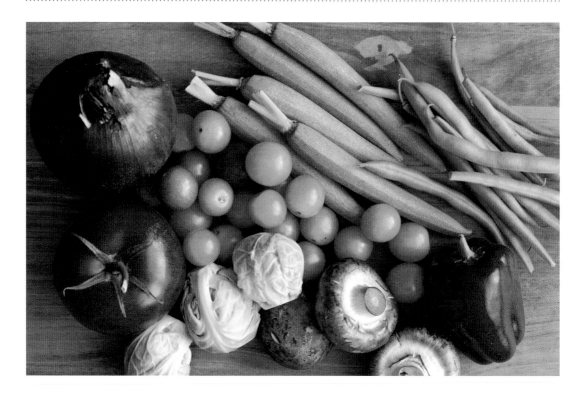

diets ate 275 to 425 calories *less* per day than those on higher energy-dense diets—even though they consumed *more* food.[23]

What's even more compelling? According to the National Weight Control Registry—a research group that's tracked more than ten thousand people who have lost weight and kept it off—eating a low-calorie, high-volume diet is one of the most important factors for success, helping dieters keep the pounds off even five years after their initial slim down.[24] Among all the people the National Weight Control Registry has studied, a whopping 98 percent reported modifying their food intake in order to lose weight.[25]

The bottom line: Eating vegetables translates into weight loss. Period. It's far more effective than drastically slashing food groups (like ditching carbs or fat) or eating a lot less of your normal foods (you'll have so little on your plate that it's a recipe for deprivation!). Research has proven it. A study in the *American Journal of Clinical Nutrition*, for example, followed ninety-seven obese women—all of whom were avoiding high-fat foods. Half were asked to increase their produce consumption, while the other half (the control group) stayed on their reduced-fat diets. At the end of one year, the women who added more vegetables lost an average of seventeen pounds—20 percent more than those just focusing on fat consumption.[26]

Then there are the benefits beyond losing weight . . .

Veggies Enhance Your Health

Nearly all veggies provide some of the fiber you need to stay satisfied. Even better, they deliver a vital dose of antioxidants (sorry, iceberg lettuce, not you). So important!

The various antioxidants in vegetables help prevent damage to your DNA—reducing your risk of heart disease, diabetes, and many types of cancer, including breast cancer. In countries where people eat a veg-rich diet, the risk of common cancers is reduced by 50 percent![27] That's why I've raised the bar from what we've known as the standard 5 a day of fruits and veg to a minimum of 5 a day from veg alone (a serving is ½ cup cooked or 1 cup raw). In fact, a minimum of 5 a day of fruits and veg is what the American Institute for Cancer Research (AICR) recommends for cancer prevention.

But remember this: Variety matters. The more colorful veggies you eat, the greater the health benefits! That's because different-colored vegetables contain different phytochemicals (there are tens of thousands of them), which add flavor, aroma, and color to foods, while helping protect your body against a host of diseases. The various phytochemicals also have a synergistic effect—which means that eating them *together* can make them more potent at disease prevention than eating them separately. That's the rainbow effect!

So go beyond your standard green veggies by adding orange carrots, red peppers, yellow squash, white asparagus, and purple eggplant. I always tell patients to treat their diet the way they would their financial portfolio—diversify! You wouldn't put everything you have into one single stock. So don't let your health ride only on romaine. Eating many kinds of fruits and veggies will deliver a broader range of health-boosting compounds that interact to protect you.

Now for the c-word.

Veggies Fight Cancer

If you want to fight one c-word, pick up another: cruciferous.

Cruciferous vegetables like broccoli contain *isothiocyanates*—compounds that trigger enzymes that neutralize and eliminate carcinogens in the body.[28] I tell patients to eat at least one serving of cruciferous vegetables from the following list per day:

- Arugula
- Bok choy
- Broccoli
- Broccoli rabeBroccoli sprouts (extremely effective!)

- Brussels sprouts
- Cabbage
- Cauliflower
- Collard or mustard greens

- Kale
- Radishes
- Turnips (roots and greens)
- Watercress

Herbs and Spices: Spice Up Your Life (Not Just Your Food)

What could be better than natural ingredients that make everything taste better without adding calories? Well, what if they also increased the nutritional value of your meals? It's true!

Take my Magical Mystery Mix (page 40), for example. It contains common turmeric, black pepper, garlic powder, and ground ginger—none of them patented or genetically engineered, all available in any supermarket, and all of which have anti-inflammatory benefits that may help fight diseases.

Turmeric has been used for medicinal purposes for ages, and promising research shows that the antioxidant curcumin in turmeric can interfere with cancer cell development and growth.[29] Other studies indicate that eating turmeric with black pepper—which contains the powerful substance piperine—improves your body's absorption of the curcumin.[30] Research

WHY YOU NEED TO *EAT* YOUR VITAMINS

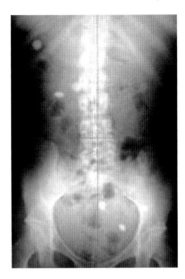

I'm frequently asked, "What about supplements? Can't you get all the nutrients you need with a daily multi?" The answer is simple: *no*. We researchers often joke that the only thing that popping excessive amounts of supplements does is make your urine more expensive. And so many people take mountains of them—and at the expense of a poor diet!

That is, if they get digested at all . . .

Check out this X-ray—I couldn't resist including it, because it's been with me for every lecture of my career and has traveled the world with me: Those white dots are whole supplements, some of which have already entered the lower G.I. tract! That means they're going out the way they came in: undigested.

Now, I do recommend certain supplements and am not entirely opposed to using them, but they're not as effective as nutrients from real food. Think of them as the cherry on top—not the entire sundae—when it comes to nutrition.

at the University of Michigan suggests that this dynamic duo can play a role in the prevention (and possibly even treatment) of breast cancer.[31]

Then there's garlic, which has long been celebrated for its ability to improve immune system function. (See, it doesn't just thwart vampires.) Garlic also contains compounds now being studied for cancer prevention.[32] Trust me: We haven't heard the end of all the amazing things garlic can do.

As for fresh herbs, many contain the same beneficial compounds as vegetables. Basil, for example, packs both antibacterial and antioxidant properties—with some evidence also linking basil with cancer prevention.[33] Another significant source of "antis" is oregano: Gram for gram, oregano contains forty-two times more antioxidant power than apples and four times more than blueberries.[34] Then there's parsley, which is so much more than a lowly restaurant plate garnish. It's rich in vitamin C and chemoprotective oils that can help eradicate certain carcinogens.[35]

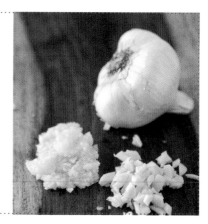

BETCHA DIDN'T KNOW: Fresh, uncooked garlic is best. Eating it this way may sound like a dare, but here's the truth: You can get more of the immunity-enhancing compound allicin in garlic when you mash or chop it and expose it to the air for a few minutes. If you can't take it that way, add chopped garlic toward the very end of cooking time to max out on flavor *and* nutrition.

I could talk for days about the health benefits of herbs and spices. So much power in such small amounts—no wonder we talk about the "spice of life."

So that's a small taste of the inside science on the veggies, herbs, and spices. Now let's flip sides for those ever-confusing proteins.

WHY I LOVE A HEALTHY DASH OF CINNAMON

We dietitians are paying more attention to cinnamon—and not just because it adds great flavor without sugar. Cinnamon contains antioxidants that research suggests can help regulate blood sugar, lower cholesterol, and even help with nausea.[36] In fact, 1 teaspoon of ground cinnamon contains as much antioxidants as a whole cup of pomegranate juice or ½ cup of blueberries!

But here's where a little knowledge goes a long way: There are two types of cinnamon sold in stores—Ceylon and cassia—and they're not created equal.

Ceylon cinnamon is known as "true cinnamon," and research suggests *that's* what you should use for one reason: It contains less coumarin. Coumarin is a blood thinning phytochemical that can cause liver damage in large amounts. Ceylon is harder to find and more expensive, but it contains far less coumarin than cassia does. Plus, it's sweeter—and you can tell your friends that you only use the "true" stuff.

my protein gps explained

I developed the Protein GPS (see pages 45 to 54) to help patients find their way through a sometimes baffling world of meats, beans, eggs, tofu, and other options—because these choices are not all created equal. The *type* of protein you choose really matters when it comes to weight loss and your health. Lean proteins like fish are just as satisfying as more fatty varieties like beef, yet usually contain far fewer calories. In fact, there's a mountain of evidence linking diets high in lean proteins to weight loss. And studies suggest the inverse to be true as well: Diets that include a lot of high-fat animal proteins cause the scale needle to go up.

The disparities in health benefits are even more dramatic: According to a recent large-scale study at the Harvard School of Public Health, eating lean proteins such as fish and beans can lower your overall risk of mortality. The same study also linked red meat consumption with a *higher* risk of mortality, as well as an increased risk for diseases such as cancer and heart disease.[37] You don't need a dietitian to tell you that's huge!

Here are a few highlights about the various proteins I recommend.

Omega-3–Rich Fish

There are so many reasons to get hooked on fish—especially fish high in omega-3s. Here are just a few of the things it can potentially do for you:[38]

- Reduce inflammation, therefore preventing a variety of conditions, from Crohn's disease to painful periods
- Prevent heart disease
- Lower blood pressure

- Increase HDL ("good") cholesterol levels and lower triglyceride levels
- May reduce the risk of developing cancer, including breast, colon, and prostate cancers
- Reduce arthritis symptoms
- Decrease dermatological disorders, such as eczema
- Protect against depression
- Improve brain function
- Potentially protect against dementia and stroke

Now, "omega-3" might sound like an evil spy agency—or the name of some distant planet—but this nutrient should be part of your world. Omega-3 is what's known as an essential fatty acid—essential because your body can't produce it. You have to *consume* essential fatty acids. There are three primary essential fatty acids to know about: docosahexaenoic acid (DHA) and eicosapentaenoic acid (EPA), which are both found in fish and other animal foods, and alpha-linolenic acid (ALA), which comes from vegetarian sources (such as flaxseeds or chia seeds).

Some of my patients get overly enthused about plant sources of omega-3s and completely avoid all meat sources of omega-3s. While I endorse includ-

> **BETCHA DIDN'T KNOW:** The gray part of your salmon may be as bad as it looks. It's primarily fat—and that's where contaminants like PCBs accumulate in farm-raised fish. So unless you know for sure that your salmon is wild, ditch the gray stuff.

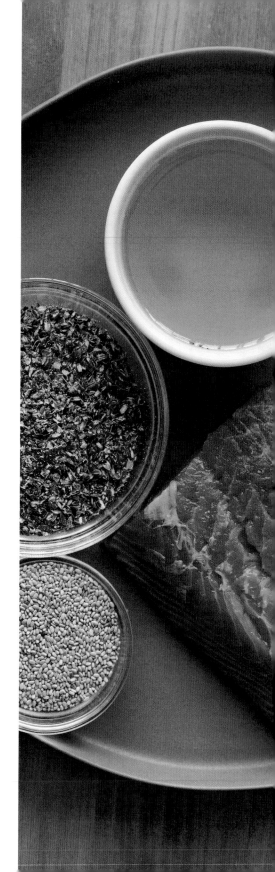

> **BETCHA DIDN'T KNOW:** Omega-3s degrade when heated—so don't overcook your fish. (The rule of thumb: ten minutes per inch of thickness.) The same can happen if you blast it over too-high heat, like with frying. Stick to steaming, broiling, baking, or grilling. Final healthy cooking tip: Eat fish together with garlic (in the same meal) to more effectively lower cholesterol.

ing the vegetarian variety in your diet, please remember that the body converts only 12 to 20 percent of the vegetarian source ALA you eat into DHA and EPA. That's it. And that's why fish plays such an important role in the nutrition plans I recommend. Fish gives you DHA and EPA in "ready to use" form.[39]

For my vegetarian-leaning patients who are willing to consider it, I recommend a fish oil supplement to compensate for the limited conversion of ALA to usable DHA and EPA. If patients avoid animal products altogether, I suggest using highly concentrated plant-based chia oil and/or flaxseed oil as part of their salad dressings to help maximize the usable form of DHA and EPA, as they can't get it from fish. In addition, I recommend microalgae oil, which contains varying amounts of DHA and EPA that can be consumed in supplement form to help obtain those valuable omega-3s.

Omega-3–rich foods also help you strike a better omega-6 balance. Let me explain: Omega-6s are polyunsaturated fatty acids found in highly refined and processed foods and vegetable oils, as well as in meat and high-fat dairy products. You do need omega-6s to produce certain hormones, help the immune system respond to injury, and enable blood clotting.[40] But too much of a good thing can have a bad effect—and most Americans get *way* too much omega-6.

Now, there's some debate about this whole "balance" issue. Many experts believe the imbalance between omega-3s and omega-6s has led to the rise of inflammation-related diseases like heart disease, cancer, and autoimmune and neurodegenerative diseases. But there's contradictory research showing that the omega-6 to omega-3 ratio does little to support your health or predict cardiovascular disease risk.[41] However, these studies have not looked at cancer or other chronic illnesses.

THE TRUTH ABOUT TILAPIA

When I was growing up, no one ever talked about tilapia. Today it's everywhere. That's because this farmed fish is inexpensive, mild, and is lower in contaminants than many ocean-grown fish. From a sustainability perspective, it's not overfished and is usually farmed conscientiously. However, there's a big catch to this big catch: Tilapia contains more omega-6 fatty acids than omega-3s. Of course, if you're at a dinner party choosing between tilapia and corn-fed steak, by all means go for the tilapia (at least it has *some* omega-3s). Just don't make tilapia your main go-to fish.

The debate aside, researchers still agree on the benefits of omega-3s in the diet. So while the jury deliberates and the research continues, my advice is that you seek out more omega-3s in your diet and eat fewer omega-6 fatty acids.

Finally, you might be wondering why I specify *wild* salmon in my recommendations. Aren't farmed salmon cheaper, more common, and just as rich in omega-3s? Yes, but studies from the Pew Foundation and the Environmental Working Group show that farmed fish sometimes have high levels of antibiotics and other toxins from their unvaried diet.[42] They may also contain higher levels of mercury and polychlorinated biphenyls (PCBs). Last I checked, you don't want any of those substances in your diet. So if you're going for salmon, go wild.

The Scoop on Soy

"Tofu or not tofu?" That is a question I've heard my entire career while working with breast cancer patients at hospitals, cancer centers, and the Beller Nutritional Institute.

Tofu and other soy products can be confusing, and the scientific studies over the last decade have only added to the puzzle: Soy can reduce the risk of breast cancer—no wait, it can't—hold on, could it actually increase your risk?

So what's the truth? Does soy protect against breast cancer or promote it?

The most recent research shows that soy either has *no* effect on breast cancer risk, or that it may actually *lower* it. According to one analysis, the estrogen-like effects of soy isoflavones are too weak to significantly affect breast tissue in healthy women—and that includes breast cancer survivors.[43] In fact, a recent large-scale study of 18,312 women found that breast cancer survivors who ate soy had a significantly reduced risk of recurrence.[44] In addition, a 2010 study published in the *Journal of Nutrition* reviewed two decades of research and concluded that soy may indeed lower the risk of breast cancer—particularly when eaten during childhood and adolescence. It may also reduce the risks of prostate cancer and heart disease and improve bone health.[45]

One reason for the contradictory research may be the *type* of soy studied. Much of the research showing a protective effect was conducted in Asian countries, where soy tends to be eaten in its traditional, unprocessed form. That's why I tell patients to stick to those types of soy, as opposed to processed products such as tofu hot dogs, which may not be as healthful.[46]

So here's my take: After reviewing hundreds of studies on soy foods and breast cancer, I believe that soy can and should be part of a healthy diet for women when eaten *in moderation* (8 to 12 ounces a week), even for those who have a prior history of breast cancer.

Why You Should Embrace the Mighty Bean

So much awesomeness in such a little package! Beans are practically a wonder food—and it's a wonder more Americans don't eat them daily!

First, let's talk weight benefits. In addition to fiber, legumes contain more protein than many other plant foods. Take a look:

1 CUP OF COOKED QUINOA = 8 GRAMS OF PROTEIN AND 5 GRAMS OF FIBER

1 CUP OF COOKED BEANS = 15 GRAMS OF PROTEIN AND 15 GRAMS OF FIBER

This high-protein, high-fiber combo causes beans to digest *slooowly,* keeping hunger at bay.[47] That may explain why bean eaters tend to have lower BMIs (Body Mass Index) and waist circumferences. The slow digestion also benefits diabetics and others who need to avoid the "blood sugar roller-coaster ride" and want long-lasting energy (basically all of us). Compelling reasons to replace typical animal proteins (chicken, turkey, beef) with beans!

Aside from being one of the best sources of fiber around, legumes such as soybeans, peas, lentils, and kidney beans may fight against cancer. They're an important source of phytochemicals, including isoflavones, a compound that may protect against cancer and heart disease, and saponins, which have been shown to help lower cholesterol.

Want proof? A study of 90,630 women by the Harvard School of Public Health found a significant link between bean and lentil consumption and a lowered risk of breast cancer, with those who ate beans most frequently (twice or more a week) enjoying the greatest benefit.[48] And a study published in the *Archives of Internal Medicine*—which tracked the health of participants over the course of nineteen years, on average—found that men and women who ate legumes four or more times a week had a 22 percent lower risk of coronary heart disease than those who ate legumes less than once a week.[49]

Beans deserve much more credit—and a bigger role in your diet.

The Sunny Side of Eggs

Eggs got a bad rap for decades. But recent evidence suggests that the old science isn't what it was cracked up to be—and that eggs actually *are* good for you in many ways.

First, and most important, eggs are rich in omega-3s—as long as you buy the kind clearly labeled "omega-3–enhanced," which contain more DHA than regular eggs. Believe me, it's worth the extra buck. They're still incredibly affordable—and eggs are also one of the highest-quality protein sources there is.

The benefits get even better: Egg yolks are the richest source of choline, a "brain food" that fights off cognitive decline. This essential nutrient also enables our cells to function properly,

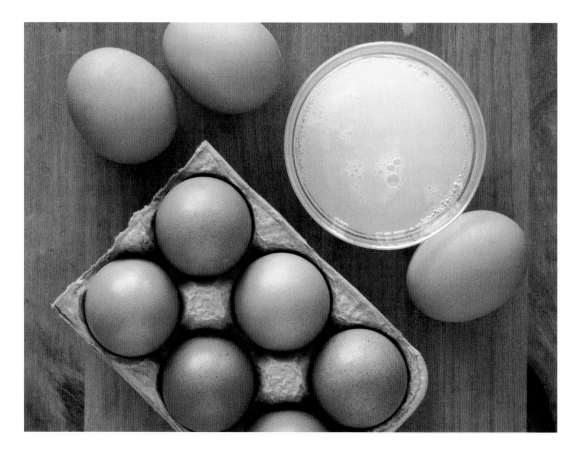

helping to transport nutrients throughout the body. And studies suggest that higher choline intake may reduce the risk of breast cancer in women, lower inflammation, and fend off other diseases and cancers, as well.[50] Yet more than 90 percent of Americans aren't getting nearly enough choline in their diets.[51] Well, now you've got an easy fix in your fridge!

Then there's the skinny factor. Studies have linked egg consumption with weight loss—thanks to all that high-quality, low-cal, sustaining protein. One study published in the *International Journal of Obesity* compared participants on an eggs-for-breakfast diet to those who ate the same number of calories worth of bagel. After eight weeks, the egg eaters had a 65 percent greater reduction in weight loss and a 34 percent greater drop in waist circumference compared to the bagel eaters. And, surprisingly, cholesterol levels didn't differ between the two groups.[52]

So what about the cholesterol controversy? Don't egg yolks contain lots of it? Yes, they do. But nutrition experts have determined that as part of an overall low-fat diet people can eat one whole egg daily without measurable changes in their blood cholesterol levels.[53] Interestingly, other studies show that it's the *saturated fat* more than the actual cholesterol in the food we eat that raises our cholesterol levels! My recommendation: In moderation, 3 to 4 yolks per week (you can have unlimited whites) can be a part of everyone's menu.

A Touch of Healthy Fats Is a Must

Nope. That's not a typo.

Despite what most people believe after all those years of fat-free faddism, we all *need* fat in our diets. Fat improves skin and hair and keeps immune systems strong. And you know what's even more surprising? Studies show that people who eat a moderate amount of *healthy* fats are more likely to stay on their diets and *lose* weight. That's because fats take longer to digest, so they keep you feeling full. They also stimulate the release of a hormone called cholecystokinin (CCK), which suppresses appetite and signals you to stop eating. But don't get excited and start putting bacon on everything—a small amount can go a long way for satiety.

And here's another good reason to add a little fat to your meals: It actually helps you absorb more of the nutrients in the foods you eat. A study at Iowa State University, for example, found that people who ate salads with a dose of fat absorbed significantly more of the lycopene and beta-carotene from the veggies than those who used fat-free dressings.[54] And recent research at Purdue University suggests that when you dress veggies with a healthy fat, such as olive oil, it takes only about 3 grams of dressing to get all the benefits from the produce. A total win-win.[55]

Again, I'm talking *moderate* amounts of fat here—about 35 grams a day, or the equivalent of 2½ tablespoons olive oil. Research suggests that limiting your intake to around this amount is key for many health reasons.

One example that's near and dear to me: I spent ten years involved in a major multicenter trial called the Women's Intervention Nutrition Study (WINS).[56] This landmark study was de-

BETCHA DIDN'T KNOW: "No smoking" applies to cooking oils, too. Smoking-hot oil can release carcinogens into the air and trigger free radicals inside of the oil. So keep temperatures low. You might not get the "extra-crispy" effect you want, but you won't get a lot of other "extras" that could hurt you either.

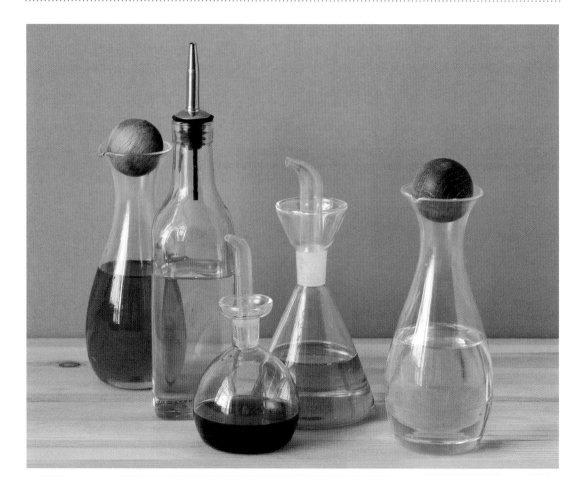

signed as a phase III prospective randomized trial, studying the effects of a low-fat diet on breast cancer recurrence. The strength of the study centered on the randomization process, which allows for the greatest reliability and validity of the study—very rare in dietary studies—and the close monitoring and control of dietary fat intake by the study participants during the trial.

The results were promising. Women in the study consumed only 30 to 35 grams of fat each day, compared to the normal recommended limit of 65 grams. These women not only experienced a decrease in weight but, most important, a decrease in breast cancer recurrence, as well. Because of these results (and the results from numerous studies linking low-fat diets to a reduced risk in other diseases), I highly recommend a low-fat diet to all my patients.[57]

The Whole Truth About Whole Grains

The term "whole grain" gets tossed around a lot, but what does it mean, exactly? And why are "enriched" and "refined" terms to avoid? Aren't those *good* words?

"Whole grain" means that all three parts of the grain kernel—the germ, bran, and endosperm—are intact, which maintains the fiber and antioxidants. So-called refined grains, on the other hand, usually have the bran and germ stripped away, leaving only the starchy endosperm. Result: You lose the fiber along with most of the antioxidants. And that's a serious loss!

The term "enriched wheat flour" (aka white flour) tells you that certain nutrients were lost during the refining process—and have been added back. However, the natural fiber can't be brought back—it can only be added in manufactured form—so the grain will never really be "whole" again.

Who cares about whole grains? Oh, just about anyone who's watching their weight.

Lots of research has linked whole grain intake with weight loss and maintenance. Researchers at Pennsylvania State University, for example, found that dieters who upped their intake of whole grains lost a higher percentage of body fat (particularly around their waistlines) over the course of the 12-week study compared to those eating refined grains.[58]

Here's why: As you know from my earlier chapters, fiber-rich whole grains keep your appetite under control so you eat less. Refined grains have the opposite effect: Your body burns through them so quickly that your blood sugar drops and—bam!—food cravings strike.

Now let's talk health. The same Penn State study also found that, in addition to weight loss, the whole grain dieters lowered their heart disease risk. That's because whole grains pack a wealth of vitamins, minerals, and hundreds of phytochemicals—all nutrients usually stripped out of refined grains. Phytochemicals protect your body's cells from damage that may lead to heart problems and other diseases like cancer.[59]

BETCHA DIDN'T KNOW: When it comes to pasta, cooking time and shape matter. In Italian, "al dente" means "to the tooth"—that the pasta has been cooked just long enough so that it still has a little chewy bite to it. And when it's prepared this way, your body has to work harder to digest it, which actually keeps your blood sugar steadier. Shaped pastas like rotini and penne are the easiest to cook al dente (compared to, say, angel hair pasta). They also scoop up more of the lycopene-rich marinara sauce.

More evidence: A review of 66 studies on whole grains found that people who consume 3 to 5 servings of whole grains a day have a 26 percent lower risk of type 2 diabetes and a 21 percent lower risk of cardiovascular disease. And they consistently weigh less over time (8 to 13 years) than those who never or rarely eat whole grains.[60]

the science behind the snacks

How Smart Snacking Keeps You From Overeating

It's the best excuse for snacking *ever*—and the best part about it? It's solidly true.

But before you go running for the pantry, let's dispel one *myth:* You know the belief that eating "mini meals" between major ones stokes your metabolism? Well, sorry, but recent research suggests that may not actually be true.[61] There's no proof that snacking keeps your metabolism running high, enabling you to burn more calories.

The real benefit of snacking? It keeps you from overeating. A ton of research shows that if you go too long without food, your blood sugar levels dip, triggering hunger—and not just for any old food, but specifically for high-sugar, high-fat items.[62] (Really, name one person who says, "Wow, I'm starving—I could sure go for some raw veg!")

Smart snacking keeps your blood sugar stable, your energy up, and your appetite in check—helping you to want less and naturally *eat* less at your next meal. A study in the journal *Appetite* found that people who ate more frequently consumed *27 percent fewer calories* during meals than those who let hours and hours pass without snacks.[63]

Granted, that stat wouldn't please parents who want their kids to clean their plates at dinner—remember being told, "Stop snacking or you'll ruin your appetite for dinner"? But it's actually a healthier approach to meals.

One exception: The midmorning snack—which is why I say it's *optional.* A recent study published in the *Journal of the American Dietetic Association* found that women who regularly allowed themselves a midmorning snack lost, on average, 7 percent of their body weight over the course of the year-long study, while those who didn't eat between breakfast and lunch did much better—losing more than 11 percent of their body weight.

What's more, the morning snackers tended to eat mindlessly, because food was simply there (oh, hello bagels in the break room!) or because they were bored (how will I survive this meeting?). It usually wasn't that they genuinely needed a caloric fix.[64] A morning snack certainly isn't a bad thing—the women in this study still lost a significant amount of weight. But the bottom line is: If you don't need it, don't eat it.

Why Portioning Is Key

Size matters when it comes to snacking. This is a key rule here!

Our whole notion of snack size has gotten completely out of hand by marketers pushing giant smoothies and bags full of "healthy" chips and trail mix. Between-meal bites have become between-meal monstrosities—with snacks now accounting for almost *one quarter* of the total calories we eat in a day.[65]

Part of that snacking insanity has to do with *how* we eat—on the go, eating straight out of a big bag or box. And research shows that that leads us to eat almost twice as much as we normally would.[66] That's why measuring and preportioning your snacks is so important. It makes the whole thing failproof.

Fruit Rules as a Snack!

I can't guarantee that an apple a day will keep the doctor away, but studies show that one will definitely keep hunger at bay. Even better? Go for an orange.

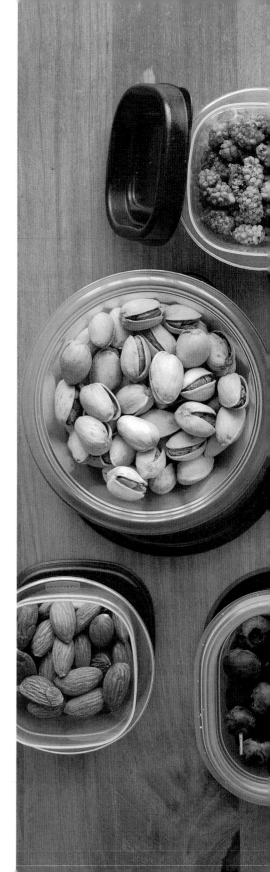

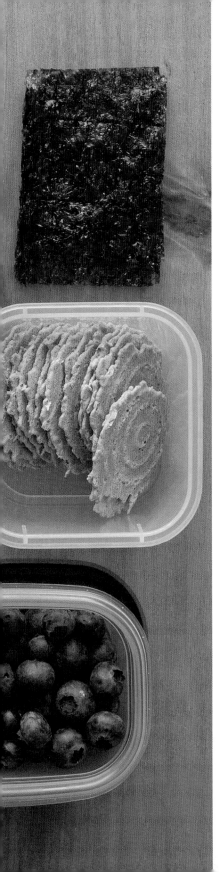

A study in the *European Journal of Clinical Nutrition* ranked thirty-eight individual items—from potatoes and cheese to cake and apples—according to their "satiety index" (how well they kept study participants from becoming hungry). Among the fruits they tested, oranges rated highest on the satiety index, followed by apples, grapes, then bananas. Fruit outranked several types of low-fiber breakfast cereals, proteins like cheese, and even brown rice in staying power.[67]

The reason? Our good friend fiber, of course! Fruit delivers a dose of fiber that will carry you through to your next meal far better than an energy bar or a typical 100-calorie snack pack.

The health benefits of fruit are also as vast as those of veggies, helping to prevent a host of diseases including heart disease, diabetes, and certain cancers. As with veggies, don't settle for monochrome: Eat a Technicolor rainbow of fruit—purple grapes, green kiwis, red berries, orange mangoes—because different fruits contain different antioxidants.

A recent study on strawberries, for example, pointed out their incredible anti-inflammatory properties, which can lower your risk for hypertention, infection, and even allergies.[68] Grapes contain a phytonutrient called resveratrol that's linked to greater longevity, as well as lowering your risk of heart disease and breast and colon cancer—and even keeping you looking younger while you're living longer![69] Fruits also work together with one another—say, when you nosh on that mixed fruit platter—to give you an even more powerful dose of antioxidants.[70]

So next time you need a snack, head for the fruit salad. If you're on the move, fruit is totally portable—that's key for me. In fact, I keep a stocked fruit bowl (tangerines and a variety of apples) on my desk for my afternoon snack and when I'm on the go. It's a far faster and healthier solution than hitting the snack machine or nearby coffee shop.

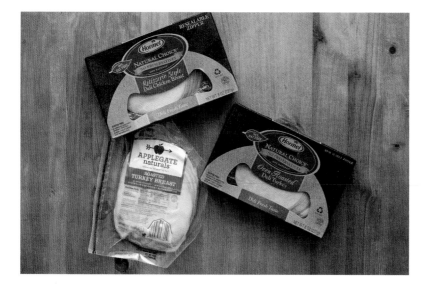

Why Should My Snacks Be Nitrate Free?

Let's say you decide to go for a half-sandwich with some turkey or sliced deli chicken as your p.m. snack.

If that's the urge, then be sure to go "nitrate free." There's some evidence that links the preservatives sodium nitrate and sodium nitrite with colon cancer. That increased risk may apply only if you consume these processed meats in very large quantities,[71] but my advice is to still take the better-safe-than-sorry approach.

Will the occasional questionable deli turkey sandwich harm you? No. As I've said before, my mantra is that it's not what you do some of the time that matters—it's what you do most of the time. But nitrates are an additive that you can, and should, live without. (If available, fresh carved is always best.)

The Trick Behind Treats

Can sweets magically cause weight loss? Keep dreaming.

But small indulgences like a piece of chocolate will keep cravings from snowballing to the point where you're eating not just one premeasured brownie but the whole pan.

In one Australian study, a group of chocolate lovers were forbidden to have even a nibble. You can guess what happened: Not only did they report strong cravings, but they became so obsessed with chocolate that they couldn't focus on anything else![72]

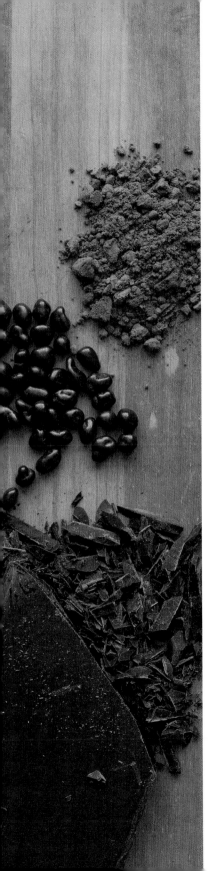

Can you believe scientists study this stuff? All they had to do was ask anyone who loves chocolate. None of us like to feel deprived! *And deprivation doesn't work anyway.* Research shows that people who have a restrictive eating style actually don't weigh any less than those who allow themselves the occasional treat.[73]

Speaking of Chocolate . . .

Those of us who love it know that it's not just another treat.

Yes, when you eat a piece of chocolate (make it dark!), you get the physical satiety from the fat it contains. But don't underestimate the *emotional satiety* you get from knowing, "Yes, I'm eating chocolate!" It literally makes you feel good. Research shows that eating chocolate can increase levels of serotonin and dopamine in your brain—two chemicals that regulate mood.[74] A happy mind and a happy belly together make better diet choices—and that's the right recipe for weight loss!

From a health perspective, cocoa is also wildly rich in antioxidants. A study at Cornell University found the antioxidant content in a cup of hot cocoa to be nearly twice as powerful as a glass of red wine, two to three times higher than a cup of green tea, and four to five times higher than black tea.[75]

As a result of all those good-for-you compounds, research has also linked dark chocolate consumption with a reduced risk of cardiovascular disease and diabetes, as well as improved immune response, cognitive function, and even protection against UV damage.[76]

Just make sure that whatever chocolate or cocoa you buy does not say "Dutch processed" or "processed with alkalai" on the label. This treatment results in a milder taste but also strips out a lot of the antioxidants. You want the real, unstripped deal—so make it at least 70 percent dark!

Once you find that dark delight, go easy—and indulge with my blessings! Sweet, huh?

notes

1. Institute of Medicine, *Dietary Reference Intakes for Energy, Carbohydrate, Fiber, Fat, Fatty Acids, Cholesterol, Protein, and Amino Acids.* Washington, D.C.: The National Academies Press; U.S. Department of Agriculture, Agricultural Research Service, 2008. Nutrient Intakes from Food: Mean Amounts Consumed per Individual, One Day, 2005–2006.

2. Wisker, E., "Metabolizable energy of diets low or high in dietary fiber from fruits or vegetables in humans." *Journal of Nutrition*, 1990, 120:1131–37.

3. Liebman, Bonnie, "Fiber Free for All: Not all fibers are equal." *Nutrition Action Newsletter*, August 1, 2008. De Koning, L., and Hu, F.B. "Do the benefits of dietary fiber extend beyond cardiovascular disease?" *Archives of Internal Medicine*, Feb. 14, 2011.

4. De Koning, L., Hu, F.B., "Do the Benefits of Dietary Fiber Extend Beyond Cardiovascular Disease?" *Archives of Internal Medicine*, Feb 14, 2011, 2.

5. Rose, D.P., et al., "High-fiber diet reduces serum estrogen concentrations in premenopausal women." *American Journal of Clinical Nutrition*, 1991 54 (3):520–25. Goldin, B.R., et al., "Estrogen excretion patterns and plasma levels in vegetarian and omnivorous women." *New England Journal of Medicine*, 1982; 307:1542–47.

6. Park, Y., et al., "Dietary fiber intake and risk of breast cancer in postmenopausal women: the National Institutes of Health-AARP Diet and Health Study." *American Journal of Clinical Nutrition*, 2009 Sep, 90(3):664–71.

7. Holmes, M.D., et al. "Dietary carbohydrates, fiber, and breast cancer risk." *American Journal of Epidemiology*, 2004 Apr 15, 159(8):732–39.

8. Chuang, S.C., et al., "Fiber intake and total and cause-specific mortality in the European Prospective Investigation into Cancer and Nutrition cohort." *American Journal of Clinical Nutrition*, 2012, 96:164–74.

9. De Koning, L., and Hu, F.B. , "Do the benefits of dietary fiber extend beyond cardiovascular disease?" *Archives of Internal Medicine*, Feb. 14, 2011. Slavin, Janice L., "Position of the American Dietetic Association: health implications of dietary fiber." *Journal of the American Dietetic Association*, 2008 Oct, 108(10):1716–31.

10. Schatzkin, et al., "Dietary fiber and whole grain consumption in relation to colorectal cancer in the NIH-AARP Diet and Health Study." *American Journal of Clinical Nutrition*, 2007 May, 85(5):1353–60. Park, Y., et al., "Dietary fiber intake and risk of colorectal cancer: a pooled analysis of prospective cohort studies." *JAMA*, 2005 Dec, 14;294 (22):2849–57.

11. Karalus, M., et al., "Fermentable fibers do not affect satiety or food intake by women who do not practice restrained eating." *Journal of the Academy of Nutrition and Dietetics*, July 9, 2012: 2212–2672.

12. Prasong, Tanmahasamut, and Liu Jingbo, "Conjugated linoleic acid blocks estrogen signaling in human breast cancer cells." *Journal of Nutrition*, March 1, 2004, vol. 134, no. 3:674–80.

13. Butler, G., and J.H. Nielsen, "Fatty acid and fat-soluble antioxidant concentrations in milk from high- and low-input conventional and organic systems: seasonal variation." *Journal of the Science of Food and Agriculture*, June 2008, volume 88, issue 8: 1431–41.

14. Report on the Food and Drug Administration's Review of the Safety of Recombinant Bovine Somatotropin; http://www.fda.gov/AnimalVeterinary/SafetyHealth/ProductSafetyInformation/ucm130321.htm

15 (1). Chan, J., "Plasma insulin-like growth factor-I and prostate cancer risk: a prospective study." *Science*, vol. 279, 563, January 23, 1998. 15 (2). Norton, A., "Blood protein linked to pancreatic cancer." *Caring 4 Cancer*, August 29, 2007.

16. Heaney, R.P., and D.A. McCarron, "Dietary changes favorably affect bone remodeling in older adults." *Journal of the American Dietetic Association*, 1999 Oct, (10):1228–33, http://www.ncbi.nlm.nih.gov/pubmed/10524386. Qin, L. Q., K., He, and J. Y. Xu, "Milk consumption and circulating insulin-like growth factor-I level: a systematic literature review." *International Journal of Food Sciences and Nutrition*, 2009, 60Suppl. 7:330–40. Epub Sept 9, 2009. Crowe, F.L., et al., "The association between diet and serum concentrations of IGF-I, IGFBP-1, IGFBP-2, and IGFBP-3 in the European Prospective Investigation into Cancer and Nutrition." *Cancer Epidemiology, Biomarkers & Prevention*, May 2009, 18(5):1333–40. Norat, T., et al., "Diet, serum insulin-like growth factor-I and IGF-binding protein-3 in European women." *European Journal of Clinical Nutrition*, Jan. 2007, 61(1):91–98. Epub Aug 9, 2006.

17. Chagas, C.E., Rogero, M.M., Martini, L.A., "Evaluating the links between intake of milk/dairy products and cancer." *Nutrition Reviews,* 2012 May, 70(5): 294–300. doi: 10.1111/j.1753-4887.2012.00464.x. Epub 2012 Mar 27. http://www.ncbi.nlm.nih.gov/pubmed/22537215

18. Shin, M.H., et al., "Intake of dairy products, calcium, and vitamin D and risk of breast cancer," *Journal of the National Cancer Institute* 94, no. 17 (2002):1301–10.

19. Danby, F.W., "Acne, dairy and cancer: The 5alpha-P link." *Dermato-Endocrinology,* 2009 Jan, 1(1):12–16.

20. Holmes, Michelle D., and Michael N. Pollak, "Dietary correlates of plasma insulin-like growth factor I and insulin-like growth factor binding protein 3 concentrations." *Cancer Epidemiology, Biomarkers & Prevention*, Sept 2002, 11, 852.

21. Weiss, D.J., and C.R. Anderton, "Determination of catechins in matcha green tea." *Journal of Chromatography A*, 2003 Sept 5, 1011(1–2):173–80.

22. Nicklas, Jacinda M., et al., "Successful Weight Loss Among Obese U.S. Adults." *American Journal of Preventive Medicine*, 2012, 42(5):481–85.

23. Ledikwe, J.H., et al., "Dietary energy density is associated with energy intake and weight status in US adults." *American Journal of Clinical Nutrition*, 2006, 83(6):1362–86.

24. Shick, S.M., Wing, R.R., Klem, M.L., McGuire, M.T., Hill, J.O., Seagle, H. "Persons successful at long-term weight loss and maintenance continue to consume a low-energy, low-fat diet." *Journal of the American Dietetic Association*, 1998 Apr, 98(4):408–13. Source: National Weight Control Registry website (www.nwcr.ws).

25. Ibid.

26. Ello-Martin, J.A., et al., "Dietary energy density in the treatment of obesity: a year-long trial comparing 2 weight-loss diets." *American Journal of Clinical Nutrition*, 2007, 85(6):1465–77.

27. Heber, David, *What Color Is Your Diet?* New York: HarperCollins (2001), p. 8.

28. Heber, D., "Vegetables, fruits and phytoestrogens in the prevention of diseases." *Journal of Postgraduate Medicine*, 2004, 50(2):145–49.

29. Aggarwal, B.B., et al., "Curcumin suppresses the paclitaxel-induced nuclear factor-kappaB pathway in breast cancer cells and inhibits lung metastasis of human breast cancer in nude mice." *Clinical Cancer Research*, 2005, 11:7490–98.

30. Srinivasan, K., "Black pepper and its pungent principle—piperine: a review of diverse physiological effects." *Crit Rev Food Sci Nutrition*, 2007, 47(8):735–48.

31. Kakarala, M., et al., "Targeting breast stem cells with the cancer preventive compounds curcumin and piperine." *Breast Cancer Research and Treatment*, 2010 Aug, 122(3):777–85. Epub Nov 7, 2009.

32. World Cancer Research Fund/American Institute for Cancer Research, *Food, Nutrition, Physical Activity, and the Prevention of Cancer: A Global Perspective.* Washington, D.C.: World Cancer Research Fund/American Institute for Cancer Research, 2007.

33. Patil, D., et al., "Antibacterial and antioxidant study of *Ocimum basilicum Labiatae* (sweet basil)." *Journal of Advanced Pharmacy Education & Research*, 2011, 2:104–12.

34. Wang, S.Y., and W. Zheng, "Antioxidant activity and phenolic compounds in selected herbs." *Journal of Agricultural and Food Chemistry*, 2001, 49(11):5165–70.

35. Pan, M.H., and C.T. Ho, "Chemopreventive effects of natural dietary compounds on cancer development." *Chemical Society Reviews*, 2008 Nov, 37(11):2558–74.

36. Ranasinghe, P., et al., "Efficacy and safety of 'true' cinnamon (*Cinnamomum zeylanicum*) as a pharmaceutical agent in diabetes: a systematic review and meta-analysis." *Pharmacognosy Research*, 2012 Apr, 4(2):73–79.

37. Pan, A., et al., "Red meat consumption and mortality: results from 2 prospective cohort studies." *Archives of Internal Medicine*, 2012, 172(7):555–63.

38. Source: Mayo Clinic.

39. Stark, A.H., et al., "Update on Alpha-Linolenic Acid." *Nutrition Reviews*, 2008, 66(6):326–32.

40. Fritsche, K., "Fatty acids as modulators of the immune response." *Annual Review of Nutrition* 26 (2006):45–73;S.

41. Griffin, B.A., "How relevant is the ratio of dietary n-6 to n-3 polyunsaturated fatty acids to cardiovascular disease risk? Evidence from the OPTILIP study." *Current Opinion in Lipidology* 19 (2008): 57–62.

42. Pew Environmental Group, "Pew Environmental Group Calls for a Crackdown on Unapproved Drug Use by Salmon Farms." 2009; available at www.pewtrusts.org (accessed June 2010).

43. Messina, M.J., and C.E. Wood, "Soy isoflavones, estrogen therapy, and breast cancer risk: analysis and commentary." *Nutrition Journal*, 2008, 7:17.

44. Nechuta, S.J., et al., "Soy food intake after diagnosis of breast cancer and survival: an in-depth analysis of combined evidence from cohort studies of US and Chinese women." *American Journal of Clinical Nutrition*, May 30, 2012.

45. Messina, M. "Insights gained from 20 years of soy research." *Journal of Nutrition*, 2010, 140 (12):2289S–95S.

46. Source: https://www.caring4cancer.com/go/cancer/nutrition/questions/soy-and-hormone-related-cancers.htm

47. McCrory, M.A., et al., "Pulse consumption, satiety, and weight management." *Advances in Nutrition*, 2010 Nov, 1(1):17–30.

48. Adebamowo, C.A., et al., "Dietary flavonols and flavonol-rich foods intake and the risk of breast cancer." *International Journal of Cancer*, 2005, 14(4):628–33.

49. Bazzano, L.A., et al., "Legume consumption and risk of coronary heart disease in US men and women NHANES I epidemiologic follow-up study." *Archives of Internal Medicine*, 2001, 161(21):2573–78.

50. Shannon, J., et al. "Food and botanical groupings and risk of breast cancer: A case-control study in Shanghai, China." *Cancer Epidemiology, Biomarkers & Prevention*, 2005, 14(1):81–90.

51. Jensen, H.H., et al., "Choline in the diets of the US population: NHANES, 2003–2004." Iowa State University (presented at Experimental Biology 2007, Washington D.C.).

52. Vander Wal, J.S., et al., "Egg breakfast enhances weight loss." *International Journal of Obesity* (London), 2008, 32(10):1545–51.

53. Fernandez, M.L., "Effects of eggs on plasma lipoproteins in healthy populations." *Food & Function*, 2010 1(2):156–60.

54. Brown, M.J., et al., "Carotenoid bioavailability is higher from salads ingested with full-fat than with fat-reduced salad dressings as measured with electrochemical detection." *American Journal of Clinical Nutrition*, 2004, 80(2):396–403.

55. Shellen, R., et al., Goltz, S.R., et al., "Meal triacylglycerol profile modulates postprandial absorption of carotenoids in humans." *Journal of Molecular Nutrition & Food Research*; 2012 Jun, 56(6):866–77.

56. Chlebowski, R.T., "Dietary fat reduction and breast cancer outcome: interim efficacy results from the Women's Intervention Nutrition Study." *Journal of the National Cancer Institute*, 2006 Dec 20, 98(24):1767–76.

57. Ibid.

58. Katcher, H.I., et al., "The effects of a whole grain-enriched hypocaloric diet on cardiovascular disease risk factors in men and women with metabolic syndrome." *American Journal of Clinical Nutrition*, 2008, 87(1):79–90.

59. Source: American Institute for Cancer Research, Caring4cancer.com

60. Ye, E.Q., et al., "Greater whole grain intake is associated with lower risk of type 2 diabetes, cardiovascular diease, and weight gain." *Journal of Nutrition*, 2012, May 30.

61. Cameron, J.D., et al., "Increased meal frequency does not promote greater weight loss in subjects who were prescribed an 8-week equi-energetic energy-restricted diet." *British Journal of Nutrition*, 2010, 103(8):1098–1101.

62. Page, K.A., et al., "Circulating glucose levels modulate neural control of desire for high-calorie foods in humans." *Journal of Clinical Investigation*, 2011, 121(10):4161–69. Dewan, S., et al., "Effects of insulin-induced hypoglycaemia on energy intake and food choice at a subsequent test meal." *Diabetes/Metabolism Research and Reviews*, 2004, 20(5):405–10.

63. Speechly, D.P., and R. Buffenstein, "Greater appetite control associated with an increased frequency of eating in lean males." *Appetite*, 1999, 33(3):285–97.

64. Kong, A., et al. "Associations between snacking and weight loss and nutrient intake among postmenopausal overweight to obese women in a dietary weight-loss intervention." *Journal of the American Dietetic Association*, 2011, 111(12):1898–1903.

65. Popkin, B.M., and C. Piernas, "Snacking increased among U.S. adults between 1977 and 2006." *Journal of Nutrition*, 2010, 140(2):325–32.

66. Wansink, Brian. *Mindless Eating: Why We Eat More Than We Think.* New York: Bantam Books (2006).

67. Holt, S.H., et al., "A satiety index of common foods." *European Journal of Clinical Nutrition*, 1995 Sep, 49(9):675–90.

68. Giampieri, F., et al., "The potential impact of strawberry on human health." *Natural Product Research*, July 13, 2012.

69. Das, D.K., et al., "Erratum to: resveratrol and red wine, healthy heart and longevity." *Heart Failure Reviews*, 2011 Jul, 16(4):425–35.

70. Liu, R.H., "Health benefits of fruit and vegetables are from additive and synergistic combinations of phytochemicals." *American Journal of Clinical Nutrition*, 2003 Sep, 78(3 Suppl):517S–520S.

71. Source: American Cancer Society. http://www.cancer.org/Cancer/News/ExpertVoices/post/2011/03/31/Hot-dog!-Headlines-Can-Be-Deceiving.aspx. Chao, A., Thun, M.J., Connell, C.J., McCullough, M.L., Jacobs, E.J., Flanders, W.D., Rodriguez, C., Sinha, R., Callê, E.E. Meat consumption and risk of colorectal cancer. *JAMA*. 2005 Jan 12, 293(2):172–82. Link to the abstract: http://www.ncbi.nlm.nih.gov/pubmed/15644544

72. Kemps, E., and M. Tiggemann, "A cognitive experimental approach to understanding and reducing food cravings." *Current Directions in Psychological Science*, 2010, 19(2)86–90.

73. McLean, J.A., and S.I. Barr, "Cognitive dietary restraint is associated with eating behaviors, lifestyle practices, personality characteristics and menstrual irregularity in college women." *Appetite*, 2003, 40(2):185–92.

74. Parker, G., et al., "Mood state effects of chocolate." *Journal of Affective Disorders*, 2006 Jun, 92(2–3):149–59.

75. Lee, K.W., et al., "Cocoa has more phenolic phytochemicals and a higher antioxidant capacity than teas and red wine." *Journal of Agricultural and Food Chemistry*, 2003 Dec 3, 51(25):7292–95.

76. Katz, D.L., et al., "Cocoa and chocolate in human health and disease." *Antioxidants & Redox Signaling*, 2011 Nov 15, 15(10):2779–81.

acknowledgments

Being surrounded with incredible people is truly the best gift, and I'm thrilled at the opportunity to express my gratitude.

To my first boss, Dr. Armando Giuliano, MD, Executive Vice Chair of Surgical Oncology at Cedars-Sinai Medical Center. In the ten years together, you've given me a wealth of knowledge both in the research and clinical patient care setting.

To Dr. Philomena McAndrew, MD, my role model for combining clinical care and deep compassion while working with oncology patients. I've learned so much during the years we've worked together. And to all the doctors and staff at Tower Hematology Oncology Medical Group, I'm so lucky to have worked with such an incredible team.

To my editor, Cassie Jones, and her assistant, Jessica McGrady. Cassie, you are a true genius at pulling everything together. I knew you got me from day one and love how you captured my fire so perfectly. I couldn't imagine doing this book with anyone else.

More thank yous to the following people at William Morrow for all your contributions and support of this book: Michael Morrison, Liate Stehlik, Lynn Grady, Tavia Kowalchuk, Joyce Wong, Ann Cahn, Lorie Pagnozzi, Karen Lumley, Sharyn Rosenblum (PR goddess), and Mary Schuck and Kris Tobiassen for your amazing creativity.

To Teri Lyn Fisher. Your stunning photographs and artistic capabilities are truly reflected throughout the pages. And to the incredible food stylist Jenny Park, thanks for always being ready to take on any challenge.

To my superstar agent, Dan Strone, CEO at Trident Media Group, and his assistant, Kseniya Zaslavskaya. Dan, you are my go-to guy across the board and invaluable to my career.

To my business consultant, Joel Fishman, who has helped me find my vision and preps me for *everything*. You make sure I'm always ready to go get 'em!

To my entertainment attorney, Ken Suddleson. Thank you for always having my best interests at heart. Your sound advice always pays off.

To Shine America and everyone at *Biggest Loser*. Lee Rierson, for believing in me and bringing me into the fold, and all the producers and amazing *BL* team members. Brandon Riegg of NBC, your enthusiasm for health and nutrition allows for a greater message on camera.

To all the reality show contestants and trainers I've had the pleasure to work with, and to all of my patients and study participants: Your quest for knowledge and weight-loss success has taught me so much and is what keeps me going. I could not have designed a winning formula without the experiences we've shared.

To Shaun Dreisbach, this book could not have come together without you. You've managed to keep me, and this project, on track—and your expertise and guidance were invaluable. And to my one-of-a-kind team at BNI! Freddy Nager, a creative genius, for always making sure I'm laughing while hard at work. Yvonne Ortega, MS, RD, CSSD, for all your impeccable fact-checking expertise. Avital Shoomer, a real go-getter, for being the best product manager. Maya Harel, your talents of managing so many aspects of BNI are beyond me. A huge thank you to Christiana Cheon—you gave your heart and soul to the project, and your contribution is immeasurable. Everyone on this project, including myself, relied on you as the go-to gal.

And to all the research assistants, project managers, and interns who are always ready for anything thrown their way: Thank you for making sure I meet deadlines and ensuring that I get home with plenty of time to play (or do homework) with my kids, a huge gift.

A sincere thanks to my friends who let me chill and give me a mental vacay from work. I always look forward to having you guys over for dinner. Best taste testers I could ask for!

TO MY GREAT BIG FAMILY: EVERY SINGLE ONE OF YOU HAD A HAND IN BRINGING ME UP AND BRINGING THIS BOOK TO FRUITION.

First and foremost, of course, my parents: My dear mother, Shula, my everything consultant, for always believing in me. You are simply and totally my best girlfriend. My forever loving father Joe, I miss you and I carry your energy with me everywhere I go. Together you've both instilled in me the "go-getter" spirit. Your accomplishments in raising four kids while working so hard, yet always making time for adventures around the world, have instilled in me a strong sense of family and the ability to work hard and play hard. You've given your only girl a passion to never settle for the ordinary.

Love you, Sheila and Lenny—you might be in-laws, but you sure don't fit the stereotype!

And to my three big brothers, Aviv, Gil, and Ron, who've toughened me up and prepped me to face any challenge. And to all my sisters-in-law, brothers-in-law, nieces, and nephews (if I named you all it would be another book). I want to thank each and every one of you. I couldn't ask for a better or bigger family.

My beautiful children—Alexia, Jonah, Keira, and Evan—what could be better than having the four of you in my life? You guys are my dream come true. You make it all worthwhile.

Best for last—Mark, my husband, my best friend, my first phone call for everything. You've truly contributed so much during the book process, from finding the latest studies to being Superdad when I had to work late. You might be a physician by trade, but everyone knows you're my #1 PR guy.

index